Point-of-Care Echocardiography

A Case-Based Visual Guide

Point-of-Care Echocardiography

A Case-Based Visual Guide

TASNEEM Z. NAQVI, MD, FRCP (UK), MMM, FASE, FACC

Professor of Medicine, Mayo College of Medicine
Consultant, Department of Cardiovascular Disease
Mayo Clinic
Scottsdale, Arizona

Contributing Editor

AFSOON FAZLINEZHAD, MD, FASE

Echocardiography Research Fellow
Mayo Clinic
Scottsdale, Arizona

ELSEVIER

Elsevier
1600 John F. Kennedy Blvd.
Ste 1800
Philadelphia, PA 19103-2899

POINT-OF-CARE ECHOCARDIOGRAPHY

ISBN: 978-0-323-61284-5

Notices

Knowledge and best practice in this field are constantly changing. As new research and experience broaden our understanding, changes in research methods, professional practices, or medical treatment may become necessary.

Practitioners and researchers must always rely on their own experience and knowledge in evaluating and using any information, methods, compounds or experiments described herein. Because of rapid advances in the medical sciences, in particular, independent verification of diagnoses and drug dosages should be made. To the fullest extent of the law, no responsibility is assumed by Elsevier, authors, editors or contributors for any injury and/or damage to persons or property as a matter of products liability, negligence or otherwise, or from any use or operation of any methods, products, instructions, or ideas contained in the material herein.

Library of Congress Control Number: 2021937543

Content Strategist: Robin Carter
Content Development Manager: Ellen Wurm-Cutter
Content Development Specialist: Casey Potter
Publishing Services Manager: Deepthi Unni
Project Manager: Janish Ashwin Paul
Design Direction: Bridget Hoette

Printed in India

Last digit is the print number: 9 8 7 6 5 4 3 2 1

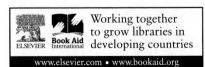

Working together
to grow libraries in
developing countries

www.elsevier.com • www.bookaid.org

Echocardiography is a powerful tool for clinical diagnosis. As technology has allowed smaller, less expensive, and more portable devices, rapid diagnosis at the bedside by healthcare providers is now possible in many clinical situations. Although auscultation with a stethoscope remains useful for some applications, such as lung sounds, numerous studies have shown that auscultation is not accurate for diagnosis of heart disease, specifically valvular heart disease, even when used by experienced healthcare providers. Instead, we can now directly image the heart in real time in patients with symptoms or a clinical presentation that might be caused by heart disease. This approach is improving patient care in the emergency department, the critical care unit, and in primary care settings. In the future, this approach may also be used to screen patient populations at risk for cardiovascular disease.

In this concise case-based book, Tasneem Naqvi provides a practical and easily understood approach to point-of-care echocardiography. Brief chapters on basic principles are clearly illustrated, including video examples, followed by detailed chapters with numerous case-based examples of different types of cardiovascular disease. The case-based approach will allow readers to quickly grasp key principles and to accelerate their point-of-care echocardiography skills.

Of course, many patients with cardiovascular disease continue to benefit from a complete diagnostic echocardiogram performed by trained sonographers and interpreted by an imaging cardiologist using a state-of-the-art echocardiography system. One of the most important attributes of a skilled healthcare professional is the ability to recognize when additional information or input from a more specialized healthcare provider is needed. The case-based approach in this book amply illustrates that principle and will enhance the reader's ability to identify which patients need referral for a more complete echocardiographic examination, as well as recognize when the point-of-care ultrasound data is adequate for clinical decision making.

Point-of-care echocardiography is a skill that is central to the practice of modern medicine. We need to ensure that healthcare providers have the training and the experience to acquire and interpret high-quality cardiac images in all patients everywhere. This book will help us achieve that goal.

Catherine M. Otto, MD
Professor of Medicine
J. Ward Kennedy-Hamilton Endowed Chair in Cardiology
Division of Cardiology
University of Washington School of Medicine
Director, Heart Valve Clinic
Associate Director, Echocardiography
University of Washington Medical Center
Seattle, Washington

May 2021

PREFACE: WHY DO WE NEED POINT-OF-CARE ECHOCARDIOGRAPHY?

The fee-for-service model in the United States healthcare system has provided highly professional, effective, and accountable patient healthcare for decades. However, the increasingly costly medical services provided to patients for their comprehensive care are no longer sustainable.

A disruption in technology began several years ago with the advent of smartphones that has enveloped itself around its consumers and has made many older technologies obsolete. These phones have now extended to wearable medical devices to monitor heart rate, heart rhythm, blood sugar, and body volume load and are bringing about a change in healthcare whereby health consumers are becoming independent and personally in charge of their health.[1]

A smartphone-sized handheld ultrasound unit first introduced by General Electric nearly a decade ago was one such disruption in healthcare. A few years later the technology has mushroomed and penetrated almost all branches of healthcare. Ultrasound transducers can now be used with smartphones and tablets, further expanding their clinical use.

The national/government healthcare systems in Europe have embraced this technology, providing most of the literature validating its sensitivity and specificity compared with a standard ultrasound system.[2] In expert hands the accuracy of handheld ultrasound devices in the detection of common cardiac findings such as left ventricular ejection fraction, wall motion, left ventricular chamber dimensions, and valve regurgitation severity or stenosis[3] when compared with standard echocardiograms remains high,[4] and significant cost savings to healthcare systems have been demonstrated.[5,6] This technology allows for a limited assessment of major findings, even in the hands of novice users. Its use reduces mortality in the ICU, reduces time to accurate diagnosis, and hence to effective treatment, even when used by medical residents.[7] It reduces the need for standard testing in as many as a third of patients and may lead to fewer ordered diagnostic tests, resulting in cost savings. It has been shown to be an effective population screening tool such as in the detection of rheumatic heart disease.[8]

Changes to the reimbursement guidelines for medical services in US healthcare support expansion of the use of this technology.[9] Medical practices and healthcare systems may reduce inefficiencies if these portable, hand-carried devices are used judiciously and by well-trained personnel.[10]

Quality and training remain essential in making effective use of these medical devices.[11] Improper use by operators with insufficient or poor training or their use outside the scope of training and practice may actually cause more harm than benefit due to suboptimal image acquisition and/or misinterpretation of findings, thus leading to misdiagnoses and inappropriate management decisions. As a result of their portable nature, these devices are being used as an extension of physical examination within a limited timeframe. Hence the users should be able to acquire focused images pertinent to patient presentation that help support, confirm, or exclude certain diagnoses that have been formulated after history, physical examination, and review of medical records and other medical tests and imaging procedures. Several societies have produced guidelines and curricula for appropriate use of this technology for their respective members.[12,13] The American Society of Echocardiography has made this subject area a high priority and is committed to being the platform on which to develop curriculum, provide training, and obtain the much-needed outcomes data for its users.

Published studies on handheld echocardiography (HHE) in cardiovasuclar medicine have either used settings simulating one of the many steps encountered in patient care[14] or have demonstrated how the use of HHE improves overall diagnostic assessment compared with standard echocardiography.[15] Other studies have demonstrated its value in reducing extra testing.[2] In fact, in the in-patient setting, use of HHE has helped in the diagnoses of as many as 76% of patients in expert hands.[10] However, the exact input the use of HHE provides during various steps in patient management in real patient care scenarios has remained unclear.

The purpose of this book is to demonstrate the use of HHE by a skilled physician during routine care of patients with simple and complex cardiovascular problems. This book comprises of a collection of HHE images obtained from real patients both during in-patient evaluations in cardiology service rounds with the cardiology team and in the out-patient setting in which HHE was used during real patient encounters. These examples illustrate how HHE can be integrated into the stepwise care of these patients. In some cases, minor edits to the patient history have been made to enhance the learning impact of each case. A focused echocardiogram was performed over 3 to 5 minutes as "a goal-oriented, limited ultrasound examination, extending physical examination."[11]

This book is also intended to discuss the clinical presentations of common cardiovascular conditions such as coronary artery disease, cardiomyopathy, heart failure, atrial fibrillation, valvular heart disease, pericardial diseases as well as diseases of the aorta. At the end of each case important current literature or professional societal guidelines have been added as a "teaching point" to bring the reader up to date on the common cardiovascular conditions encountered in today's cardiology practice.

We hope this book will spark an interest among other physicians, students, and trainees to improve their personal skills in performing echocardiography to effectively use it in their daily clinical practices.

I am grateful to our patients without whom this book would not be possible and to my family members who supported me in devoting countless hours to this book.

Practical demonstration of HHE systems used in this book, use of HHE in a volunteer, didactic lectures on topics covered in this book and more case examples interested readers may explore a virtual course on HHE 16.

Tasneem Z. Naqvi, MD

References

1. Chamsi-Pasha MA, Sengupta PP, Zoghbi WA. Handheld echocardiography current state and future perspectives. *Circulation*. 2017;136:2178-2188.
2. Cardim N, Dalen H, Voigt JU, et al. The use of handheld ultrasound devices: a position statement of the European Association of Cardiovascular Imaging (2018 update). *Eur Heart J Cardiovasc Imaging*. 2019;20:245-252.
3. Thomas F, Flint N, Setareh-Shenas S, Rader F, Kobal SL, Siegel RJ. Accuracy and efficacy of hand-held echocardiography in diagnosing valve disease: a systematic review. *Am J Med*. 2018;131:1155-1160.
4. Prinz C, Voigt JU. Diagnostic accuracy of a handheld ultrasound scanner in routine patients referred for echocardiography. *J Am Soc Echocardiogr*. 2011;24:111-1116.
5. Galasko GI, Barnes SC, Collinson P, Lahiri A, Senior R. What is the most cost-effective strategy to screen for left ventricular systolic dysfunction: natriuretic peptides, the electrocardiogram, hand-held echocardiography, traditional echocardiography, or their combination? *Eur Heart J*. 2006;27:193-200.
6. Cardim N, Golfin CF, Ferreira D, et al. Usefulness of a new miniaturized echocardiographic system in outpatient cardiology consultations as an extension of physical examination. *J Am Soc Echocardiogr*. 2011;24:117-124.
7. Razi R, Estrada JR, Doll J, Spencer KT. Bedside hand-carried ultrasound by internal medicine residents versus traditional clinical assessment for the identification of systolic dysfunction in patients admitted with decompensated heart failure. *J Am Soc Echocardiogr*. 2011;24:1319-1324.
8. Beaton A, Lu JC, Aliku T, et al. The utility of handheld echocardiography for early rheumatic heart disease diagnosis: a field study. *Eur Heart J Cardiovasc Imaging*. 2015;16:475-482.

9. https://info.hapusa.com/blog-0/medicare-proposed-major-cut-in-radiology-reimbursement-for-2021.

10. Di Bello V, Carrubba SL, Conte L. Incremental value of pocket-sized echocardiography in addition to physical examination during inpatient cardiology evaluation: a multicenter Italian study (SIEC). *Echocardiography.* 2015;32:1463-1470.

11. Sicari R, Galderisi M, Voigt JU, Habib G, Zamorano JL, Lancellotti P, Badano LP. The use of pocket-size imaging devices: a position statement of the European Association of Echocardiography. *Eur J Echocardiogr.* 2011;12:85-87.

12. Galusko V, Bodger O, Ionescu A. A systematic review of pocket-sized imaging devices: small and mighty? *Echo Res Pract.* 2018;5:4:113-138.

13. Melamed R, Sprenkle MD, Ulstad VK, et al. Assessment of left ventricular function by intensivists using hand-held echocardiography. *Chest.* 2009;135:1416-1420.

14. Mehta M, Jacobson T, Peters D, et al. Handheld ultrasound versus physical examination in patients referred for transthoracic echocardiography for a suspected cardiac condition. *J Am Coll Cardiol Img.* 2014;7:983-990.

15. Khan HA, Wineinger NE, Uddin PQ, Mehta HS, Rubenson DS, Topol EJ. Can hospital rounds with pocket ultrasound by cardiologists reduce standard echocardiography? *Am J Med.* 2014;127:669.

16. https://ce.mayo.edu/pocechoonline

CONTENTS

Abbreviations: HHE hand-held echocardiography RA, right atrium; RV, right ventricle PA, pulmonary artery IVS, interventricular septum, Ao, aortic root PLAX: parasternal long-axis, LA: left atrium, TTE: transthoracic echocardiogram

Cardiovascular Anatomy and Physiology Review

CHAPTER 1

Cardiac Anatomy

Cardiac Chambers

A normal human heart is located in the center of the chest cavity and comprises of 4 chambers: two smaller chambers on top, called the left atrium and the right atrium, and two larger and more muscular chambers below, called the left ventricle (LV) and the right ventricle (RV). The left and right sides of the heart are separated by a curtain-like partition that separates the left and right atria, called the interatrial septum, and a predominantly muscular partition that separates the left and right ventricles, called the interventricular septum (Fig. 1.1).

The right ventricle receives deoxygenated blood from the body via the superior vena cava (SVC) and the inferior vena cava (IVC), and the right atrium (RA) ejects it into the pulmonary artery. The left ventricle receives oxygenated blood through the pulmonary veins and the left atrium and ejects it into the body through the aorta (Fig. 1.2).

The RV has thinner walls than the LV. This is because the RV pumps blood into a low-pressure pulmonary arterial system, whereas the LV generates higher pressures and has thicker walls because it ejects blood into a higher-pressure arterial system or the systemic circulation through the aorta. Oxygen is extracted from blood in each organ, and the deoxygenated blood then enters the right atrium. The SVC receives deoxygenated blood from the head, neck, upper extremities, and the thoracic (chest) cavity, whereas the IVC receives deoxygenated blood from the lower extremities and organs present in the belly, such as the stomach, large intestines, small intestines, kidneys, spleen, liver, and genital organs. This blood goes through the RA into the RV, which then pumps this deoxygenated or venous (blue) blood into the lungs. The blood is oxygenated here and returned to the left side of the heart through the pulmonary veins into the LA (red); and ultimately to the LV, which then ejects it into the aorta (Fig. 1.3).

As a result of its embryologic development that involves rotation and looping, the heart is rotated on an axis so that the right-sided chambers (the RA, RV, and pulmonary artery) are oriented anteriorly and the left-sided structures (the LA, LV, and aorta) are posterior in orientation (Fig. 1.4).

Cardiac Valves

The LA and the LV are separated by a valve called the mitral valve, and the RA and the RV are separated by a valve called the tricuspid valve. These valves open in diastole to allow for filling of the ventricles by the atria and close in systole to prevent the back flow of blood into the atria as the left and right ventricles contract to eject blood into the aorta and the pulmonary artery, respectively. The mitral valve has two leaflets, anterior and posterior, whereas the tricuspid valve has three leaflets (Fig. 1.4).

An additional two valves, called the semilunar valves, separate the ventricles from the aorta and the pulmonary artery. These are called the aortic valve (located between the left ventricle and the aorta) and the pulmonary valve (located between the right ventricle and the pulmonary artery). These valves each have three leaflets (or cusps) (Fig. 1.4).

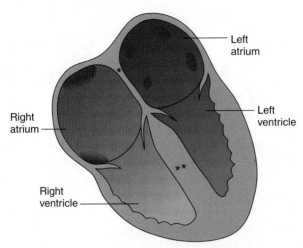

Fig. 1.1 Four Cardiac Chambers. Interatrial septum separates left and right atria (single black asterisk), and interventricular septum separates left and right ventricles (double black asterisks). *LA*, left atrium; *LV*, left ventricle; *RA*, right atrium; *RV*, right ventricle. (Used with permission of the Mayo Foundation for Medical Education and Research. All rights reserved.)

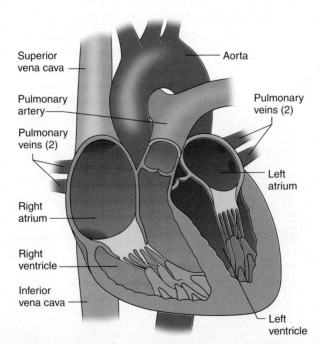

Fig. 1.2 Cardiac Chambers' Venous and Arterial Connections. Venous connections to the right atrium are the superior and inferior vena cavae. Venous connections to the left atrium are the left and right pulmonary veins (there are normally four pulmonary veins, two from the left lung, two from the right lung). The pulmonary artery arises from the right ventricle, and the aorta arises from the left ventricle. (Used with permission of the Mayo Foundation for Medical Education and Research. All rights reserved.)

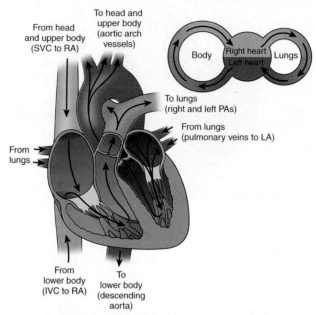

Fig. 1.3 Direction of Blood Flow Into the Cardiac Chambers. Venous blood is shown in blue and arterial blood in red. Deoxygenated blood from the superior vena cava (SVC) and the inferior vena cava (IVC) enters the right atrium (RA), the right ventricle (RV), and the pulmonary artery (PA). Oxygenated blood from the lungs enters the left atrium (LA) through the four pulmonary veins, then into the left ventricle (LV) and the aorta. The cartoon on the right depicts the venous and arterial circulations. Arrows indicate the direction of blood flow. (Used with permission of the Mayo Foundation for Medical Education and Research. All rights reserved.)

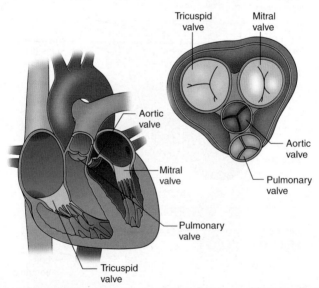

Fig. 1.4 Anterior Location of Pulmonary Artery Compared With Aorta (Left and Right Panels). Atrioventricular valves separate the atria from the ventricles: mitral valve on the left side, and tricuspid valve on the right side. The semilunar valves separate the ventricles from the great vessels: aortic valve on the left side, and pulmonary valve on the right side (left panel). The mitral valve has two leaflets: anterior and posterior leaflets. The tricuspid valve (as the name indicates) has three leaflets: septal, anterior, and posterior leaflets. The aortic and pulmonary valves each have three leaflets (or cusps) (right panel). (Used with permission of the Mayo Foundation for Medical Education and Research. All rights reserved.)

CHAPTER 2

Cardiac Vascular Connections, Anatomy, and Ultrasound Imaging

Major Blood Vessels Encountered During Routine Echocardiography

Aorta

It arises from the left ventricle and is divided into the aortic root, tubular ascending aorta, aortic arch, descending thoracic aorta, and abdominal aorta (Fig. 2.1). All these aortic segments are assessed during routine echocardiography.

The tubular ascending aorta comprises of a proximal portion, from the sinotubular junction to the pulmonary artery level, and a distal portion, from the pulmonary artery to the origin of the brachiocephalic artery (Fig. 2.1). The aortic arch gives rise to three major branches, the brachiocephalic or innominate artery, the left common carotid artery, and the left subclavian artery; and then continues as the descending thoracic aorta (Fig. 2.1). The aortic arch is the segment between the brachiocephalic artery and the left subclavian artery. Below the diaphragm, the aorta continues as the abdominal aorta.

The descending thoracic aorta has a proximal segment, from the left subclavian artery to the pulmonary artery, and a distal segment, from the pulmonary artery to the diaphragm (Fig. 2.1). The abdominal aorta is divided into a proximal segment, from the diaphragm to the renal arteries (suprarenal aorta), and a distal segment, from the renal arteries to the iliac bifurcation (infrarenal segment) (Fig. 2.1).

The celiac and superior mesenteric arteries that supply blood to the stomach, spleen, pancreas, and intestines arise from the suprarenal aorta and the inferior mesenteric artery that supplies the kidneys and lower portion of the intestines arises from the infrarenal aorta. The aorta then divides into the two common iliac arteries. The external iliac artery continues below the origin of the left and right renal arteries as the femoral artery on either side and supplies blood to the lower extremities. The presence of an aortic aneurysm can be evaluated during routine echocardiography and are most commonly located in the infrarenal portion of the abdominal aorta.

Ultrasound Imaging of Cardiac Vascular Connections

AORTA

Ultrasound imaging of the aorta is performed using various imaging windows along its course (Fig. 2.2). The aortic root and ascending aorta are readily visualized during routine parasternal imaging (Fig. 2.3). The aortic root comprises of the aortic annulus, aortic valve, aortic sinuses, and sinotubular junction. The ascending aorta often requires a higher imaging window (one or two intercostal spaces higher) than the aortic root; otherwise, enlargement of this segment of the

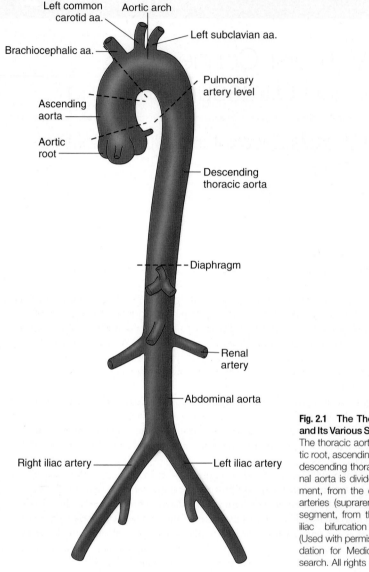

Fig. 2.1 The Thoracoabdominal Aorta and Its Various Sections and Branches. The thoracic aorta comprises of the aortic root, ascending aorta, aortic arch, and descending thoracic aorta. The abdominal aorta is divided into a proximal segment, from the diaphragm to the renal arteries (suprarenal aorta), and a distal segment, from the renal arteries to the iliac bifurcation (infrarenal segment). (Used with permission of the Mayo Foundation for Medical Education and Research. All rights reserved.)

aorta can be missed (Fig. 2.4). The aortic root and ascending aorta should also be visualized from the right parasternal window when an aortic root, ascending aorta, or aortic valve pathology is suspected (Fig. 2.5). The aortic arch and proximal descending thoracic aorta are visualized from the sternal notch at the base of the neck (Fig. 2.6).

Aortic dimensions are routinely measured at the aortic sinuses and ascending aorta. The mid portion of the descending thoracic aorta can be routinely visualized posterior to the LA in the parasternal long axis (PLAX) view (Fig. 2.3) and lateral to the LA in the apical 4-chamber view. The distal portion of the descending aorta can be visualized in the off-axis 2-chamber view.

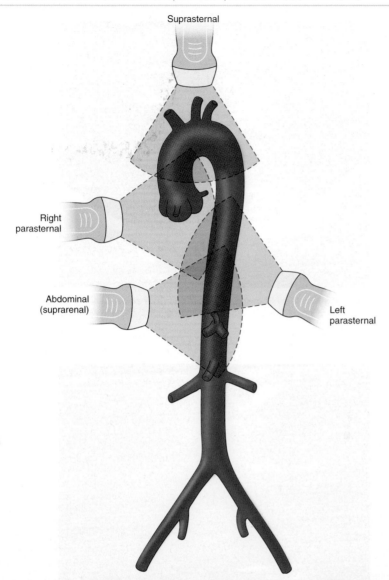

Fig. 2.2 The Echocardiographic Imaging Planes Used to Visualize Different Segments of the Aorta. (Used with permission of the Mayo Foundation for Medical Education and Research. All rights reserved.)

The abdominal aorta lies posterior and to the left of the inferior vena cava and is imaged from the subcostal window in the short- and long-axis views and is able to demonstrate normal anatomy (Fig. 2.7), aortic enlargement, aortic dissection flap, and aortic atheroma (Fig. 2.8).

PULMONARY ARTERY

It arises from the right ventricle and is located anterior to the aortic root and ascending aorta. It divides into right and left pulmonary arteries for the right and left lungs, respectively. The right pulmonary artery crosses posterior to the distal ascending aorta.

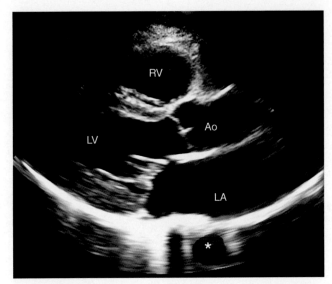

Fig. 2.3 **Parasternal Long-Axis View Showing Normal Aortic Root and Ascending Aorta.** The thoracic aorta (*) lies behind the left atrium. *Ao,* Aortic root and ascending aorta; *LA,* left atrium; *LV,* left ventricle; *RV, right ventricle.*

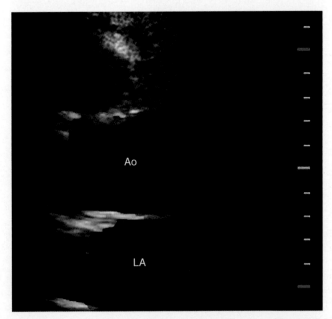

Fig. 2.4 **Parasternal Long-Axis View Showing Dilated Mid-Ascending Aorta Measuring 4.5 cm.** *Ao,* Mid-ascending aorta; *LA,* left atrium.

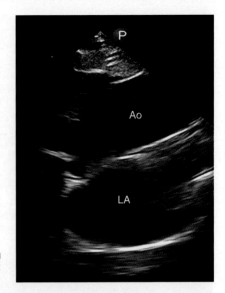

Fig. 2.5 Right Parasternal Long-Axis View Showing Dilated Mid-Ascending Aorta. *Ao,* Mid-ascending aorta; *LA,* left atrium.

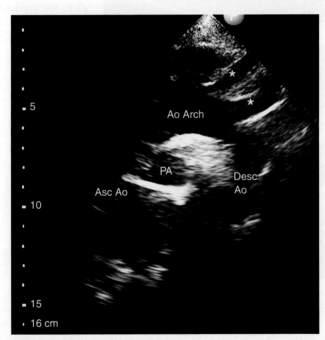

Fig. 2.6 Aortic arch (Ao arch); arch vessels (white asterisks): ascending aorta (Asc Ao) and proximal descending aorta (Desc Ao) visualized from the sternal notch at the base of the neck. *PA,* Pulmonary artery.

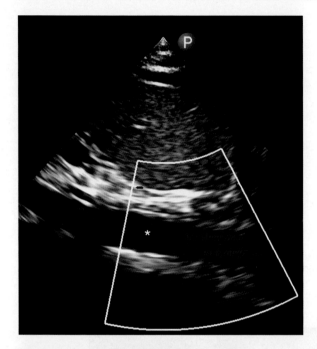

Fig. 2.7 Normal Abdominal Aorta (*) in the Long-Axis View With Color Doppler.

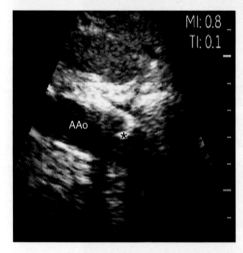

Fig. 2.8 Abdominal Aorta (AAo) in the Long-Axis View Showing Protruding Atheroma (Black Asterisk).

The main pulmonary artery and the right pulmonary artery can be routinely visualized from the short-axis view of the base of the heart (Fig. 2.9) and from the sternal notch where they are seen below the aortic arch (Fig. 2.10). The main pulmonary artery, its bifurcation, and right and left pulmonary arteries can also be visualized from the subcostal view.

INFERIOR VENA CAVA (IVC)

It is a large vein, which brings deoxygenated blood from the lower half of the body, and enters the right atrium from below.

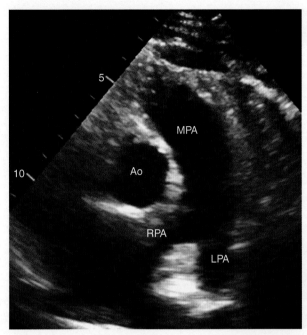

Fig. 2.9 Parasternal Short-Axis View Showing Main Pulmonary Artery (MPA) Bifurcating Into Right (RPA) and Left Pulmonary Arteries (LPA). Image acquired using a standard ultrasound platform. *Ao,* Ascending aorta.

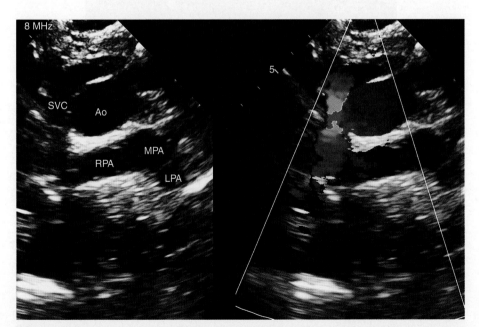

Fig. 2.10 Suprasternal Views, Two-Dimensional (2D) on the Left and Color Doppler on the Right Showing Main Pulmonary Artery (MPA) Bifurcating Into Right (RPA) and Left Pulmonary Arteries (LPA). Image acquired using a standard ultrasound platform. *Ao,* Aortic arch; *SVC,* superior vena cava.

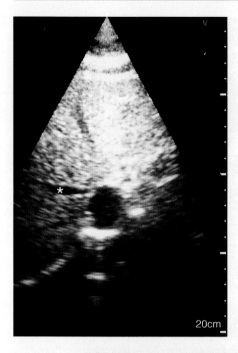

Fig. 2.11 Subcostal View Showing Collapsed Small Inferior Vena Cava (IVC: White Asterisk) in a Patient With Hypovolemia.

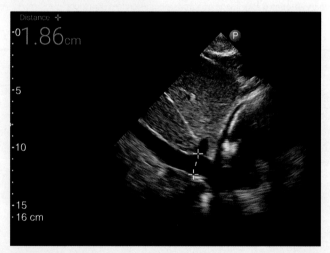

Fig. 2.12 Subcostal View Showing Normal-Sized Inferior Vena Cava Measuring 1.86 cm at Expiratory Phase of Respiration.

The IVC can be visualized from the subcostal window (Figs. 2.11, 2.12, and 2.13A and B) and the transhepatic view, if epigastric imaging is not feasible. Right atrial pressure is measured by the size of the IVC and decrease in its diameter with inspiration or sniffing as shown in Table 2.1.

Two-dimensional (2D) assessment of hepatic veins and color Doppler flow in the hepatic vein can be used to assess hepatic venous congestion caused by elevation of right heart pressures. Reversal of systolic color Doppler flow in the hepatic veins indicates severe tricuspid regurgitation.

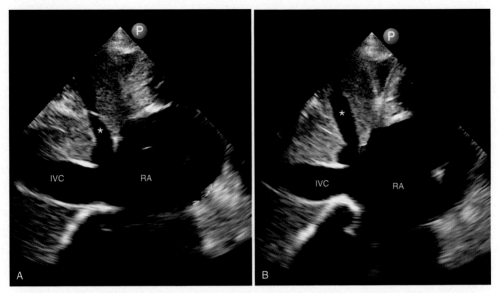

Fig. 2.13 (A) Subcostal view, showing a dilated inferior vena cava (IVC) and hepatic vein (white asterisk). (B) Subcostal view in the same patient, showing minimal inspiratory collapse of the inferior vena cava (IVC). *RA,* Right atrium.

TABLE 2.1 ■ **Estimation of Right Atrium Pressure on the Basis of Inferior Vena Cava Diameter and Collapse**

Variables	Normal [0-5 (3) mm Hg]	Intermediate [5-10 (8) mm Hg]	High (15 mm Hg)
Inferior vena cava diameter	≤21 mm	≤21 mm; >21 mm	>21 mm
Collapse with sniff	>50%	<50%; >50%	<50%

From Rudski, LG, Lai, WW, Afilalo, J, et al. Guidelines for the echocardiographic assessment of the right heart in adults: a report from the American Society of Echocardiography. Endorsed by the European Association of Echocardiography, a registered branch of the European Society of Cardiology, and the Canadian Society of Echocardiography. *J Am Soc Echocardiogr.* 2010;23:685–713.

CORONARY SINUS

It carries deoxygenated blood from the heart, it encircles the heart, and it is c-shaped. It is located within the atrioventricular groove along with the left circumflex coronary artery, and it enters the right atrium, where the blood it carries mixes with deoxygenated blood from the rest of the body.

The coronary sinus may be visualized in the PLAX view or the foreshortened apical 4-chamber view and is most easily visualized in the RV inflow view (Fig. 2.14).

The upper right and left pulmonary veins can be visualized in the apical 4-chamber view, with an anterior tilt of the transducer (Fig. 2.15). The descending thoracic aorta lies lateral to the left atrium in this view.

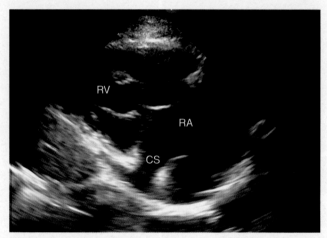

Fig. 2.14 Parasternal Right Ventricular Inflow View Showing a Dilated Coronary Sinus (CS). *RA,* Right atrium; *RV,* right ventricle.

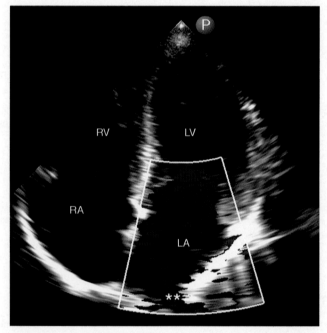

Fig. 2.15 Apical 4-Chamber View Showing Left Upper Pulmonary Venous Doppler Inflow (Double White Asterisks). *LA,* Left atrium; *LV,* left ventricle; *RA,* right atrium; *RV,* right ventricle.

SUPERIOR VENA CAVA (SVC)

It is a large vein, which brings deoxygenated blood from the top half of the body, and enters the right atrium from above.

The SVC can be visualized from the suprasternal and supraclavicular windows (Fig. 2.10).

CORONARY ARTERIES

The left coronary artery arises from the left coronary sinus and the right coronary artery from the right coronary sinus.

The left coronary artery divides into the left anterior descending and the left circumflex coronary arteries that supply the anterior and lateral walls of the left ventricle. The right coronary artery supplies the right ventricle and inferior portion of the heart. These may be visualized arising from the aortic sinuses in the short-axis view of the aortic root.

Aortic Imaging in Disease

When assessing dilation of the ascending aorta at the level of the aortic sinuses, the ascending aorta can be shown in conventional parasternal views (Figs. 2.4 and 2.5) and in apical views (Fig. 2.16).

Aortic dissection and an aneurysmal aortic root in the ascending aorta can be visualized in the parasternal views. Dissection extending to or originating in the thoracic aorta can be visualized in suprasternal (Fig. 2.17) and abdominal aortic imaging views.

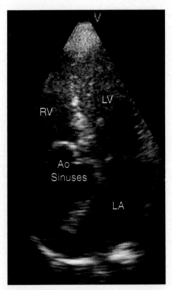

Fig. 2.16 Apical 5-Chamber View Showing Dilated Aortic Sinuses (Ao Sinuses). *LA,* Left atrium; *LV,* left ventricle; *RV,* right ventricle.

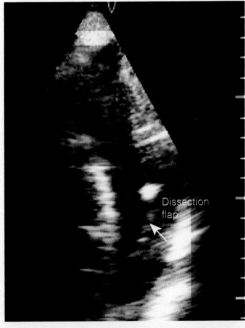

Fig. 2.17 Suprasternal View Showing Dissection Flap (white linear line) Originating at the Level of the Subclavian Artery.

References

Rudski, LG, Lai, WW, Afilalo, J, et al. Guidelines for the echocardiographic assessment of the right heart in adults: a report from the American Society of Echocardiography. Endorsed by the European Association of Echocardiography, a registered branch of the European Society of Cardiology, and the Canadian Society of Echocardiography. *J Am Soc Echocardiogr.* 2010;23:685–713.

CHAPTER 3

Cardiac Physiology

Cardiac Cycle

The cardiac cycle comprises of a systolic phase and a diastolic phase. The systolic phase is comprised of an isovolumic contraction phase, during which the pressure in the ventricles rises until it becomes greater than the pressure in the great artery into which the blood is to be ejected, at which point the semilunar valves open. As the name indicates (isovolumic), there is no change in ventricular volume during this phase. Next is an ejection phase, during which the ventricles continue to contract and eject blood into the aorta and the pulmonary artery. A drop in ventricular pressure during the end of ejection makes the semilunar valves close (when the aortic pressure exceeds the left ventricular pressure or the pulmonary artery pressure exceeds the right ventricular pressure). The diastolic phase is comprised of an isovolumic relaxation phase, during which the pressure in the ventricles falls until it becomes lower than the pressure in the atria: the isovolumetric relaxation phase. Again, as the name indicates (isovolumic), there is no change in ventricular volume during this phase. This phase ends with the opening of the mitral valve on the left side and the tricuspid valve on the right, as the ongoing ventricular relaxation causes lowering of the ventricular pressures compared with the atrial pressures and allowing filling of the ventricles from the atria. The filling phase ends when the ventricular pressures become higher than the atrial pressures, the mitral valve closes on the left side, and the tricuspid valve closes on the right side.

The left and right atria fill with venous blood from the pulmonary veins and the superior and inferior vena cavae, respectively, throughout the cardiac cycle and only eject blood into the ventricles late during the diastolic phase of the cardiac cycle (after the "P" wave on the ECG), contributing to the late diastolic filling of the ventricles. The systolic and diastolic phases cause a pressure-volume relationship during the cardiac cycle (Fig. 3.1).

EJECTION FRACTION AND CARDIAC OUTPUT

It is important to distinguish between ejection fraction and cardiac output (Fig. 3.2). Stroke volume (in mL or cc) is the actual amount of blood ejected from the ventricles with each cardiac cycle. Stroke volume multiplied by heart rate per minute is the cardiac output (liters/min).

Figure 3.3A shows examples of normal cardiac output and normal ejection fraction (EF); Figure 3.3B shows decreased EF and normal cardiac output as in dilated ischemic or nonischemic cardiomyopathy; Figure 3.3C shows normal EF with decreased cardiac output as in restrictive cardiomyopathy.

The usual cause of a low EF is impairment of ventricular contraction, although increased afterload as well as preload may also reduce EF. Reduced EF of the left and right ventricles may occur as a result of damage to the heart muscle from conditions such as a myocardial infarction (from blockage of blood flow to the heart muscle) causing necrosis of the heart muscle, inflammation or infection of the heart muscle, and hereditary or genetic heart muscle disorders, as well as from abnormal loading conditions, such as obstruction (anatomic or physiologic) to the forward flow of blood or incomplete duration of ejection, such as in tachyarrhythmias.

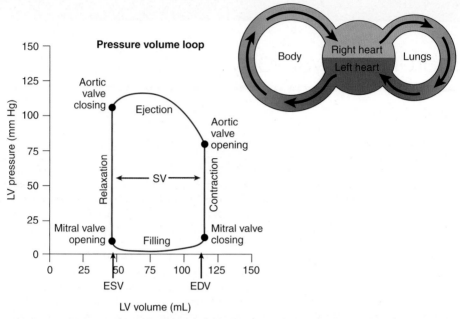

Fig. 3.1 Normal left and right ventricles eject approximately 60% of the blood these chambers receive during the diastolic phase of the cardiac cycle into the aorta and pulmonary artery, respectively. Ejection of less than 55% of blood into the great vessels with a cardiac cycle is considered abnormal. (Used with permission of the Mayo Foundation for Medical Education and Research. All rights reserved.)

Left ventricular ejection fraction (LVEF)

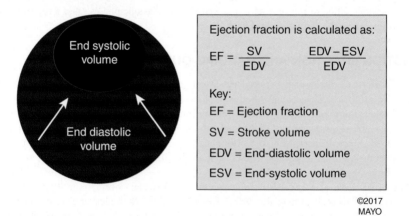

Ejection fraction is calculated as:

$$EF = \frac{SV}{EDV} \qquad \frac{EDV - ESV}{EDV}$$

Key:

EF = Ejection fraction

SV = Stroke volume

EDV = End-diastolic volume

ESV = End-systolic volume

©2017
MAYO

Fig. 3.2 Ejection fraction (as the name indicates) is the percentage of end diastolic volume of blood that is ejected out of the ventricles with each cardiac cycle. (Used with permission of the Mayo Foundation for Medical Education and Research. All rights reserved.)

Ejection fraction and stroke volume

A = Normal ejection fraction and stroke volume
B = Normal stroke volume, low ejection fraction
C = Low stroke volume, but normal ejection fraction

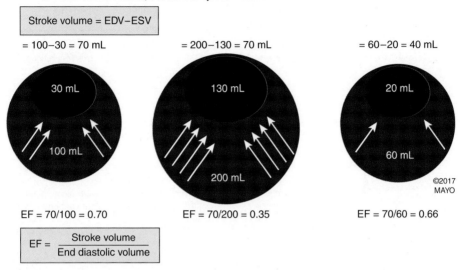

Stroke volume = EDV−ESV

= 100−30 = 70 mL   = 200−130 = 70 mL   = 60−20 = 40 mL

30 mL   130 mL   20 mL

100 mL   200 mL   60 mL

©2017 MAYO

EF = 70/100 = 0.70   EF = 70/200 = 0.35   EF = 70/60 = 0.66

$$EF = \frac{Stroke\ volume}{End\ diastolic\ volume}$$

Fig. 3.3 A normal ejection fraction and stroke volume (A), decreased ejection fraction and normal stroke volume (B), and normal ejection fraction with decreased stroke volume (C) examples are shown. (Used with permission of the Mayo Foundation for Medical Education and Research. All rights reserved.)

EF is being replaced by other more accurate methods of assessment of ventricular contraction, most notably, speckle-tracking strain imaging. A low stroke volume may occur because of a low EF and conditions such as valve dysfunction, tachyarrhythmias, intracardiac shunting, volume depletion, and increased afterload. A reduced EF or a reduced stroke volume may lead to neurohormonal adaptation in the body, leading to salt and water retention and development of congestive heart failure. The progressive stages of left ventricular systolic dysfunction are shown in Table 3.1.

Abnormalities of cardiac rhythm—in particular, atrial flutter and atrial fibrillation—impair the ability of the atria to contract and relax, thereby reducing the late contribution to the ventricular diastolic filling, and hence reducing the amount of blood the ventricles eject in the systolic phase. They also simultaneously cause congestion in the pulmonary circulation and decreased cardiac output. Poor contraction and relaxation of the atria causes atrial enlargement, and stasis of blood in the atria increases the risk for blood clot formation in the atria.

Conditions that increase the work of the left ventricle, such as high blood pressure or aortic stenosis, lead to a concentric increase in left ventricular muscle wall thickness with normal left ventricular cavity size—(called *concentric remodelling*) or in a more advanced form (left ventricular hypertrophy), when an increase in wall thickness is associated with cavity dilation. Conditions such as long-standing hypertension, diabetes mellitus, and coronary artery disease (obstruction of the blood supply to the heart by abnormal plaque formation in the coronary arteries), and other diseases of the heart muscle cause an increase in collagen content in the left ventricle, making it less compliant. Increased muscle thickness and development of fibrosis lead to impairment of the diastolic filling of the left ventricle.

Progressive stages of diastolic dysfunction are shown in Table 3.2.

TABLE 3.1 ■ Normal Left Ventricular Ejection Fraction and Common Causes and Symptoms Associated With Various Grades of Abnormal Left Ventricular Ejection Fraction

Left Ventricular Ejection Fraction	Definition	Conditions	Diastolic Function	Symptoms
Normal	≥55%	Healthy adults	Normal	None
Mildly abnormal	40%-54%	Hypertension; diabetes; coronary artery disease (CAD); genetic, viral and postpartum cardiomyopathy; early stages of infiltrative cardiomyopathy	Normal or mildly abnormal	Dyspnea on exertion, fatigue, palpitations
Moderately abnormal	30%-39%	Ischemic and nonischemic cardiomyopathy	Usually abnormal	Dyspnea on minimal exertion, fatigue, palpitations, ankle edema
Severely abnormal	<30%	Ischemic and nonischemic cardiomyopathy, restrictive cardiomyopathy, infiltrative cardiomyopathy	Abnormal	Heart failure, hospitalizations, need for defibrillator with or without biventricular pacemaker

TABLE 3.2 ■ Normal Left Ventricular Diastolic Function and Common Causes and Symptoms Associated With Various Grades of Abnormal Left Ventricular Diastolic Function

Diastolic Function Grade	Left Ventricular Diastolic Pressure	Conditions	Left Ventricular Ejection Fraction	Symptoms
Normal	Normal	Healthy adults	Normal	None
Mildly abnormal	Normal	Hypertension, diabetes, coronary artery disease (CAD), obesity	Usually normal	Dyspnea on moderate exertion
Moderately abnormal	Elevated	End-stage renal disease, CAD, ischemic and nonischemic cardiomyopathy	Normal or reduced	Dyspnea on minimal exertion
Severely abnormal	Markedly elevated	End-stage renal disease, infiltrative cardiomyopathy, ischemic and nonischemic cardiomyopathy	Borderline normal or reduced	Dyspnea at rest

Handheld Echocardiography Devices and Cardiac Imaging Techniques

CHAPTER 4

Handheld Echocardiographic Devices and Imaging Features

Similar to the miniaturization of computers, ultrasound systems have also been miniaturized with improving technology. These devices can be hand-carried and, more recently, handheld. The first handheld device, Vscan, was introduced by General Electric (Milwaukee, USA) in 2012. In 2017, Vscan Extend was introduced. Newer technology comprises of various ultrasound transducers that can be connected to Android or iOS devices or both. These include: Lumify (Philips, USA) that allows connecting an ultrasound transducer to an Android tablet was introduced in 2017. Newer devices from other vendors have become available, including Butterfly iQ (Butterfly, USA), that uses chip technology instead of piezoelectric crystals, enabling a single probe to be in a linear, curved, or phased array format.

Wireless units such as SonoQue (O2 Lifecare, USA) compatible with iOS technology, and Vscan air (GE Healthcare) compatible with Android and iOS phones and tablets. Kosmos platform is a new patented transducer with AI technology compatible with Android tablets which guides the operator on probe orientation, detects adequacy of image quality and has pulsed wave (PW) and continuous wave (CW) Doppler besides color Doppler. Vscan Extend is a smartphone-like ultrasound device with either the choice of an inbuilt cardiac or cardiac and vascular transducer. Newer handheld devices comprise of a transducer attached to an Android or iOS device or to both. All the newer devices allow for digital entry of patients' demographics. Images can be stored in the hard drive and transferred to an external device or sent/stored via web browser with the newer devices. Examination logs are stored as consecutive numbers, along with the date the examination was performed. Each examination folder has still images, cine loops, and color Doppler loops. Lumify and Butterfly iQ allow for M-mode measurements besides two-dimensional (2D) and color Doppler imaging, which are available in all devices. The measure function includes linear dimensions and area. PW (SonoQue and Kosmos) and CW (Cosmos) is becoming available in the most recent devices.

During an ultrasound examination, the device is held in the palm of one hand and the ultrasound transducer is held with the opposite hand to image the patient. All controls can be manipulated with either the left or right thumb. These include selection of the type of imaging modality (cardiac, vascular, or abdominal), creating a new patient or searching the image directory, color Doppler modality, and image store setting in either a still-image or cine-loop format. The device, smartphone, or tablet, may be placed on the bed or the patient's body if needed and feasible.

The differences between handheld echocardiographs and standard echocardiographs are detailed in Table 4.1.

TABLE 4.1 ■ Comparison Between Handheld and Standard Echocardiographs

Features	Handheld Echocardiographs	Standard Echocardiographs
Modality	Pocket-size system used as an extension of physical examination	Large platforms used to acquire images separate from physician evaluation
Operator	Usually a physician	Usually a sonographer
Training	Limited to extensive, depending on user	Extensive
Capabilities	Limited evaluation to answer a major clinical question	Can do limited and comprehensive evaluation of heart, valves, and blood vessels
Portability	Immediately available for cardiac emergencies	Bedside imaging modality, but some delay in machine boot up and imaging
Examination duration	2-10 min per study, battery operated, allows few focused exams	15-60 min per study, electric power operated
Number of images	Limited, average 5	Extensive, average 100
Impact on decision making	Instantaneous if performed by a skilled operator who is also involved in patient care	Multiple personnel involved in performing and reviewing imaging studies who are usually not directly involved in patient care in the US. Inherent delay in the final report.
Image quality	Good	Excellent
Color Doppler	Available, fixed aliasing velocity	Available, can change aliasing velocity
CW and PW Doppler	Yes, in most recent devices only	Yes
3D imaging	No	Yes
Imaging sector width	Limited (up to 70 degrees)	Wide-sector width (10-120 degrees)
Compatibility with other devices	Individual units or can be plugged with Android and Apple smartphones and tablets	Stand-alone platforms
Cost	$2,000-$10,000	$90,000-$400,000
Gain	Can adjust overall gain	Can adjust overall and TGC gain
Tissue Doppler and Strain	No	Yes, can evaluate subclinical cardiac dysfunction and dyssynchrony
Diastolic function and filling pressures	SonoQue and Kosmos	Comprehensive assessment possible
Pulmonary artery pressure	Kosmos only at present	Yes
Depth	Can adjust depth to 24 cm	Can adjust depth up to 50 cm for typical cardiac transducer
Focus	Not available in most devices	Focusing available to improve visualization of target structures
Vendors	Five and increasing	Several
Transducers	Cardiac and vascular	Multiple cardiac and vascular
Valve stenosis quantitation	Visual assessment and planimetry	Quantitation available by Doppler, 2D, and 3D planimetry

Continued

TABLE 4.1 ■ **Comparison Between Handheld and Standard Echocardiographs** (Continued)

Features	Handheld Echocardiographs	Standard Echocardiographs
Valve regurgitation quantitation	Visual	Quantitation by Doppler, 2D, and 3D
LVEF quantitation	Visual	Available by 2D and 3D
Imaging storage	Limited	Extensive in the servers
Reporting	No	Extensive
Billing	No	Yes, multiple billing codes
Comparison from prior	Limited	Multiple studies can be compared
Calculation	Limited to linear dimensions and area	Comprehensive calculation package
Live remote viewing of images	Possible in newer devices	Yes

2D, Two-dimensional; *3D,* three-dimensional; *CW,* continuous wave; *LVEF,* left ventricular ejection fraction; *PW,* pulsed wave; *TGC,* time gain compensation; *US,* ultrasound.

CHAPTER 5

How to Perform Ultrasound of the Heart and Its Arterial and Venous Connections

Patient Positioning

- Semi-recumbent position on the left side with the head elevated
- Left arm under the head or the pillow
- Right arm on the right side

Operator Positioning

Right-handed operator: The operator sits on the patient's right side with the transducer in the right hand and uses the left hand to operate the ultrasound system.

Left-handed operator: The operator sits on the patient's left side facing the patient with transducer in the left hand and uses the right hand to operate the ultrasound system.

Echocardiographic Windows

Standard imaging windows used in transthoracic echocardiography are: (1) parasternal, (2) apical, (3) subcostal, and (4) suprasternal (Fig. 5.1). From each imaging window, several different imaging views can be further obtained.

Echocardiographic Imaging Planes

The basic imaging planes are sagittal, coronal, and transverse. The sagittal plane bisects the heart longitudinally from the anterior to the posterior plane. It is used to visualize the heart in the parasternal long-axis and apical 2- and 3-chamber views. The transverse plane bisects the heart horizontally and is used to visualize the heart in the short axis at the base, mid, and apical regions. The coronal plane bisects the heart longitudinally from the apex to the aortic valve and is used to visualize the heart in the 4- and 5-chamber views (Fig. 5.2).

Imaging Transducer Motion

To evaluate a complex 3-dimensional (3D) organ, such as the heart using single-plane imaging of 2-dimensional (2D) imaging systems, several transducer motions are performed to allow for multiplane cardiac imaging (Fig. 5.3) as follows:

- *Sliding* refers to relocating the transducer on the skin's surface; it is the process of physically moving the point of contact between the transducer and the skin from one imaging window to another.

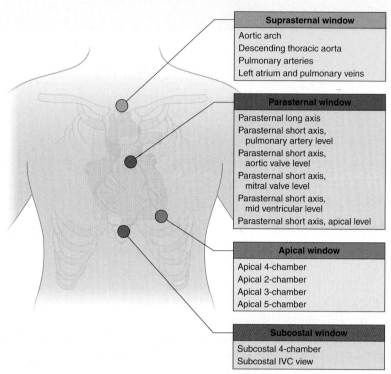

Suprasternal window
Aortic arch
Descending thoracic aorta
Pulmonary arteries
Left atrium and pulmonary veins

Parasternal window
Parasternal long axis
Parasternal short axis, pulmonary artery level
Parasternal short axis, aortic valve level
Parasternal short axis, mitral valve level
Parasternal short axis, mid ventricular level
Parasternal short axis, apical level

Apical window
Apical 4-chamber
Apical 2-chamber
Apical 3-chamber
Apical 5-chamber

Subcostal window
Subcostal 4-chamber
Subcostal IVC view

Fig. 5.1   Standard Imaging Windows Used in Transthoracic Imaging. *IVC,* Inferior vena cava.

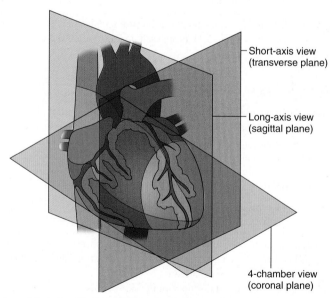

Short-axis view
(transverse plane)

Long-axis view
(sagittal plane)

4-chamber view
(coronal plane)

Fig. 5.2   Ultrasound Imaging Planes: Sagittal, Coronal, and Transverse. (From Soni NJ, Arntfield R, Kory P. *Point-of-Care Ultrasound.* Philadelphia, PA: Elsevier/Saunders; 2015.)

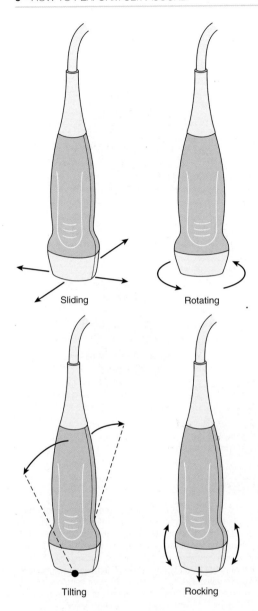

Sliding

Rotating

Tilting

Rocking

Fig. 5.3 Types of Ultrasound Transducer Motion to Allow for Multiplane Cardiac Imaging. (From Soni NJ, Arntfield R, Kory P. *Point-of-Care Ultrasound.* Philadelphia, PA: Elsevier/Saunders; 2015.)

- *Rotating* refers to twisting the transducer on its central axis, like a corkscrew. Clockwise rotation by 40–70 degrees from the sagittal plane used to obtain the parasternal long-axis view allows imaging of the heart in the transverse plane, and counterclockwise rotation of the transducer by 50–90 degrees from the 4-chamber plane (coronal plane) allows visualization of the heart in the 2-chamber and 3-chamber planes (sagittal planes).
- *Tilting*, also called sweeping, fanning, or angling, refers to changing the angle of the imaging plane while maintaining the point of contact with the skin's surface. This "cross-plane" movement allows the provider to sweep through a structure of interest from left to right, superior to inferior, or anterior to posterior (Fig. 5.4).

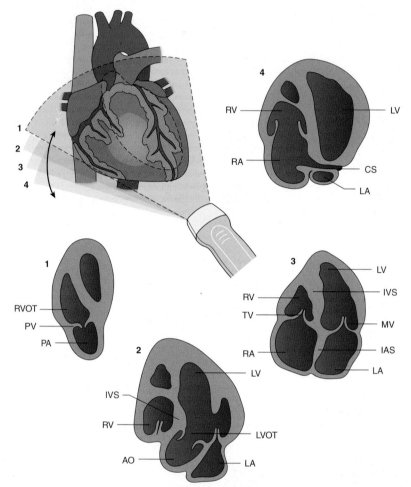

Fig. 5.4 Anteroposterior cardiac sweep from the apical 4-chamber view by anteroposterior tilting motion of the transducer to visualize structures from the most anterior plane (right ventricular outflow tract, pulmonic valve, pulmonary artery) to the anterior plane (aortic valve, left ventricular outflow tract), mid plane (true 4-chamber view showing the right and left ventricle and right and left atria in the longest length), and posterior plane (coronary sinus, posterior portions of the atria and ventricles). *AO,* Aorta; *CS,* coronary sinus; *IAS,* interatrial septum; *IVS,* interventricular septum; *LA,* left atrium; *LV,* left ventricle; *LVOT,* left ventricular outflow tract; *MV,* mitral valve; *PA,* pulmonary artery; *PV,* pulmonic valve; *RA,* right atrium; *RV,* right ventricle; *RVOT,* right ventricular outflow tract; *TV,* tricuspid valve. (From Mitchell C, Rahko PS, Blauwet LA, Canaday B, Finstuen JA, Foster MC, Horton K, Ogunyankin KO, Palma RA, Velazquez EJ. Guidelines for performing a comprehensive transthoracic echocardiographic examination in adults: Recommendations from the American Society of Echocardiography. *J Am Soc Echocardiogr.* 2019;32(1):1–64. doi:10.1016/j.echo. 2018.06.004. Epub 2018 Oct 1. PMID: 30282592.)

- *Rocking* refers to aiming the ultrasound beam either toward or away from the transducer orientation marker, or notch, while maintaining the point of contact with the skin's surface. This "in-plane" movement allows centering of the image on the screen without changing the imaging plane and allows visualization beyond the current field of view in a specific direction.

Parasternal Imaging

LONG-AXIS IMAGING

- Transducer position is at the left sternal edge, from the second to the fourth intercostal (IC) space (Fig. 5.5, Video 5.1).
- Transducer marker direction points toward the right shoulder.
- From the same transducer position, tilting the transducer anteriorly shows the long axis of the right ventricle (RV), the tricuspid valve, and the right atrium (RV inflow view); and tilting the transducer upward and toward the left shoulder shows the RV outflow tract, the pulmonic valve, and the pulmonary artery (RV outflow view).

SHORT-AXIS IMAGING

- Transducer position is the same as the parasternal long axis (PLAX).
- It requires a 40–70 degree clockwise rotation from the PLAX view so that the marker dot direction points toward the left shoulder (Fig. 5.6, Video 5.2)
- The axis of the transducer is between the right hip and the left shoulder.
- An upward-to-downward tilting of the transducer from the same acoustic window allows visualization of serial cross-sectional images from the cardiac base to apex to acquire serial parasternal short-axis views.

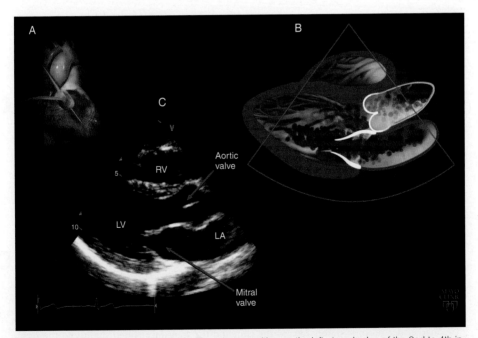

Fig. 5.5 Parasternal Long-Axis View. (A) Transducer position on the left sternal edge of the 2nd to 4th intercostal space and imaging plane. (B) Cross-sectional anatomy. (C) Parasternal long-axis ultrasound view. *LA*, Left atrium; *LV*, left ventricle; *RV*, right ventricle. (Used with permission of the Mayo Foundation for Medical Education and Research. All rights reserved.)

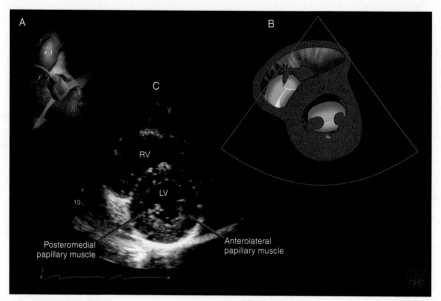

Fig. 5.6   Parasternal Short-Axis View at the Mid-Ventricular Level. A 40- to 70-degree clockwise rotation from the PLAX with the marker dot direction pointing toward the left shoulder. (A) Imaging plane. (B) Cross-sectional anatomy. (C) Parasternal mid-ventricular short-axis ultrasound view. *LV,* Left ventricle; *RV,* right ventricle. (Used with permission of the Mayo Foundation for Medical Education and Research. All rights reserved.)

APICAL IMAGING

- Transducer is slid toward the apical impulse of the heart.
- Transducer marker orientation toward the right shoulder, and the transducer marker direction unchanged allows for visualization of the 4-chamber view of the left heart on the left side and the right heart on the right side of the image display (Fig. 5.7, Video 5.3). If the transducer is rotated so that the marker position is pointing toward the ground, the cardiac orientation is switched so the left heart is on the right side and right heart is on the left side on the image display.
- The apical 2-chamber view is obtained by a 60-degree counterclockwise rotation of the transducer.
- An additional 60-degree counterclockwise rotation from the 2-chamber view gives the 3-chamber view.

SUBCOSTAL IMAGING

- Transducer is positioned horizontally under the xiphisternum (Fig. 5.8, Video 5.4).
- Marker dot position is toward the left shoulder.
- Patient is supine with head flat and knees bent to relax the abdomen. Inspiratory breath hold is often required to visualize the subcostal 4-chamber view.
- A 90-degree counterclockwise rotation from the subcostal 4-chamber view so that the marker dot position points toward the chin and the transducer tilted slightly to the right allows for visualization of the inferior vena cava (IVC) in its long-axis plane.
- Tilting the transducer to the left allows for visualization of the abdominal aorta in its long-axis plane.

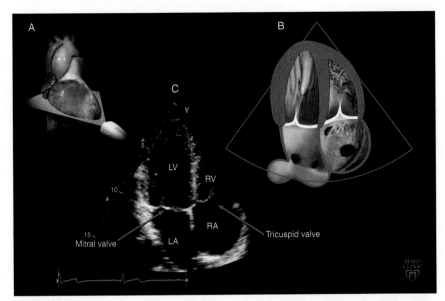

Fig. 5.7 Apical 4-Chamber View. (A) Transducer position at the cardiac apex and imaging plane. (B) Cross-sectional anatomy. (C) Apical 4-chamber ultrasound view. *LA,* Left atrium; *RA,* right atrium; *LV,* left ventricle; *RV,* right ventricle. (Used with permission of the Mayo Foundation for Medical Education and Research. All rights reserved.)

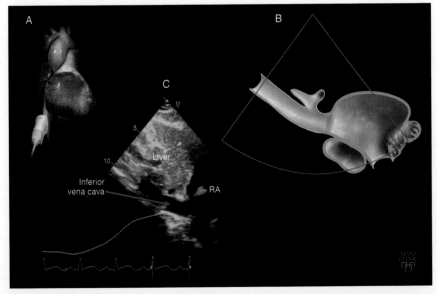

Fig. 5.8 Inferior Vena Cava View. Subcostal imaging from the xiphisternum with the subject laying supine, head flat, and knees bent to relax the abdomen. Transducer is placed horizontally at the xiphisternum, with the marker dot position toward the left shoulder. Inspiratory breath hold is often required to visualize the subcostal 4-chamber view. There is a 90-degree clockwise rotation from the subcostal 4-chamber view so that the marker dot position pointing toward the chin provides a sagittal view of the inferior vena cava. (A) Transducer position and imaging plane. (B) Cross-sectional anatomy. (C) Longitudinal ultrasound view of the inferior vena cava. *RA,* Right atrium. (Used with permission of the Mayo Foundation for Medical Education and Research. All rights reserved.)

SUPRASTERNAL IMAGING

- Transducer position in the suprasternal notch (Figs. 5.1 and 2.6).
- Patient is supine with the neck hyperextended. The head is rotated slightly toward the left.
- Marker dot position points toward the left jaw.
- This allows for visualization of the aortic arch, the great vessels originating from the aortic arch, and the proximal thoracic aorta. A slight clockwise rotation and anterior tilt shows the distal ascending aorta.
- A 90-degree rotation and rightward tilt shows the superior vena cava (SVC) (Fig. 2.10).

CHAPTER 6

Normal Echocardiogram

Using the imaging technique described in Chapter 5, a series of images obtained in normal adults using handheld echocardiogram devices are shown in Figs. 6.1–6.11 and in Videos 6.1–6.11. ▶

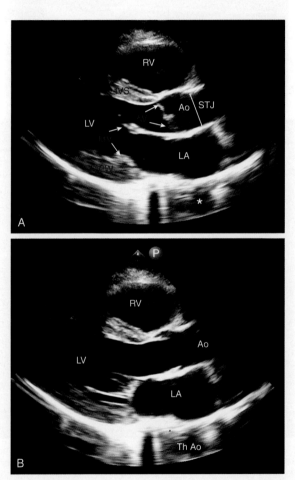

Fig. 6.1 Parasternal long-axis (PLAX) view in diastole (A) and systole (B) showing from anterior to posterior: normal right ventricle (RV) outflow tract (RV), normal interventricular septum (IVS), normal left ventricular (LV) cavity size, normal LV posterior wall (PW) and thickness, and no pericardial effusion. The aortic (AV) and mitral (MV) valves appear normal, as is the aortic root size at the sinuses (Ao), the sinotubular junction (STJ), and the left atrium (LA). The mitral valve opens in diastole and the aortic valve in systole. The descending thoracic aorta (white asterisk in A, Th Ao in B) is the most posterior structure behind the left atrium and is normal in size.

33

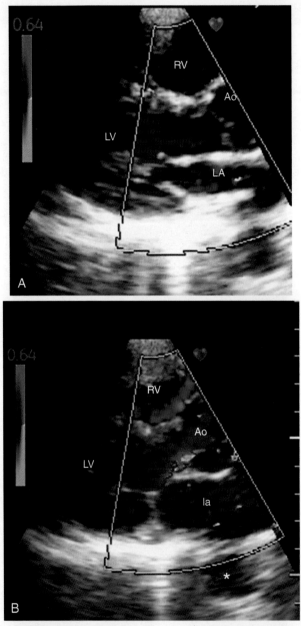

Fig. 6.2 (A) PLAX view with color Doppler in diastole showing a closed normal aortic valve and an open mitral valve with no aortic regurgitation. Blood flow toward the transducer is depicted as red-orange and away as blue. Note the aliasing velocity scale on the left set at 0.64 cm/s. Normal color Doppler velocity scale should be set to ≥60 cm/s. Lower color Doppler scale will falsely increase the regurgitant and stenotic color flow. (B) Shows the systolic phase of the cardiac cycle with an open aortic valve. Blood flow going through the aortic valve is indicated in orange color, because the blood flow is toward the transducer. Note the closed mitral valve without regurgitation. *Ao,* Aorta; *LA,* left atrium; *LV,* left ventricle, *RV,* right ventricle.

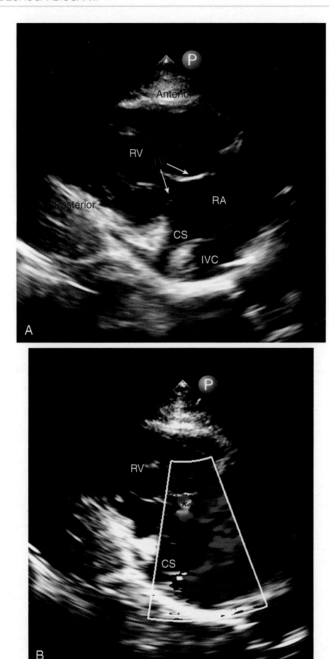

Fig. 6.3 (A) Shows a two-dimensional (2D) right ventricular inflow view with anterior and posterior right ventricular walls, RV cavity, anterior and posterior leaflets of the tricuspid valve, coronary sinus (CS), and the inferior vena cava (IVC) entry into the right atrium (RA). (B) Shows the right ventricular inflow view with color Doppler. The red color in the RA is the inferior vena cava IVC flow into it. The small blue color Doppler on the atrial side of the tricuspid valve (white asterisk in B) is the trace tricuspid regurgitation seen in many normal adults. Blood flow toward the transducer is depicted as red and away as blue. *CS,* Coronary sinus; *RV,* right ventricle.

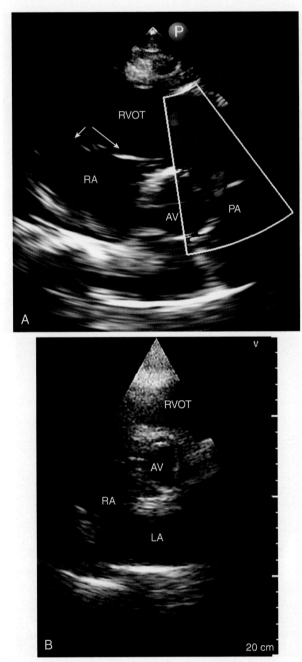

Fig. 6.4 A Parasternal Short-Axis (PSAX) View at the Basal Cardiac Level in the Diastolic Phase of the Cardiac Cycle. (A) Shown from right to left are the pulmonic valve with mild pulmonic valve insufficiency (white asterisk in the orange jet in A, the aortic valve (AV), and the tricuspid valve between RA and RVOT; and from anterior to posterior are the right ventricular outflow tract (RVOT), the aortic valve (AV), and the left atrium (LA) (B). The aliasing velocity scale is set at 0.60 m/s (B) Shows the same view in systole. The AV is in the center, is open, and has three cusps. *LA,* Left atrium; *PA,* pulmonary artery; *RA,* right atrium; *RVOT,* right ventricular outflow tract.

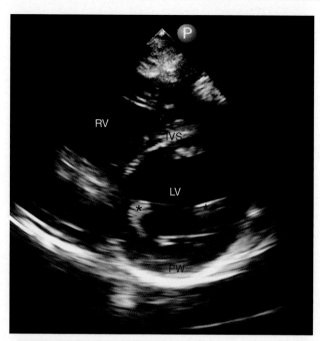

Fig. 6.5 A parasternal short-axis (PSAX) view at the mid-papillary muscle level in diastole showing from anterior to posterior: normal RV size, normal interventricular septal (IVS) thickness, normal LV cavity size, normal LV posterior wall (PW) and thickness, and no pericardial effusion. Anterolateral and posteromedial papillary muscles are shown in red asterisks. *RV,* Right ventricle; *LV,* left ventricle.

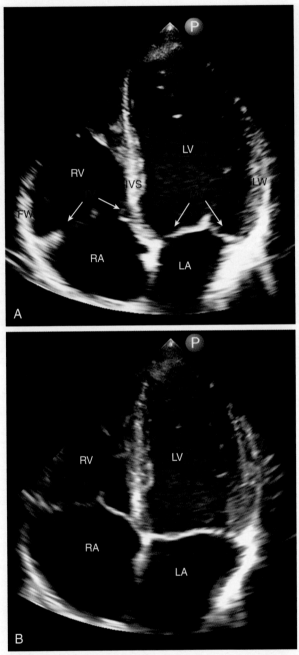

Fig. 6.6 Apical 4-chamber view in diastole (A) and systole (B). Four cardiac chambers—left ventricle (LV), right ventricle (RV), left atrium (LA), and right atrium (RA)—are seen. The mitral valve in the left heart and tricuspid valve in the right heart are seen. The lateral wall (LW) of the LV, the interventricular septum (IVS), and the RV free wall are seen.

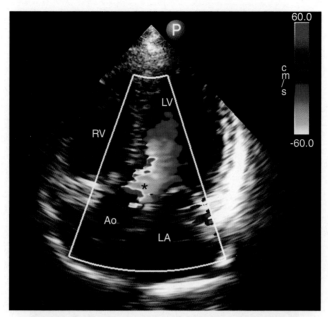

Fig. 6.7 Apical 5-chamber view with color Doppler showing normal laminar flow across the left ventricular outflow tract. Note the aliasing velocity scale on the right set at 0.60 m/s. *Ao,* Aortic root; *LA,* left atrium; *LV,* left ventricle; *RV,* right ventricle.

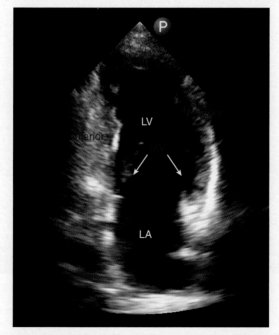

Fig. 6.8 Two-chamber view in diastole showing a normal left ventricle (LV), left atrium (LA), and mitral valve. The anterior and inferior walls of the LV are seen.

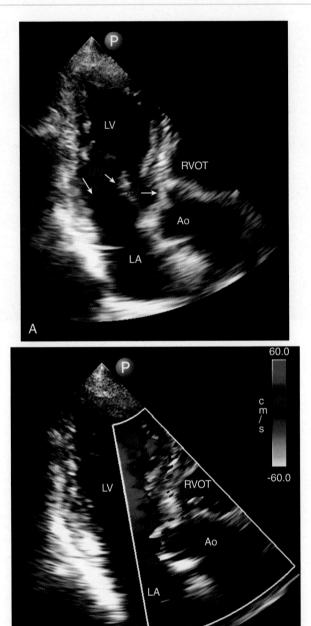

Fig. 6.9   Apical 3-chamber view in two-dimensional (2D) (A) and color Doppler (B). Normal left ventricle, left atrium, aortic and mitral valves, aortic root, and part of the right ventricle are shown. The anterior interventricular septum and LV posterior wall are seen. Aortic and mitral valves appear normal as do the aortic root size at the sinuses, the sinotubular junction, and the left atrium. No aortic regurgitation is seen in B across a closed aortic valve, and forward flow in orange is seen entering the LV across the mitral valve. A trivial jet of pulmonic regurgitation is shown by the red color near the RV outflow tract. Note the aliasing velocity scale on the right set at 0.60 cm/s. *Ao,* Aortic root; *LA,* left atrium; *LV,* left ventricle; *RVOT,* right ventricular outflow tract.

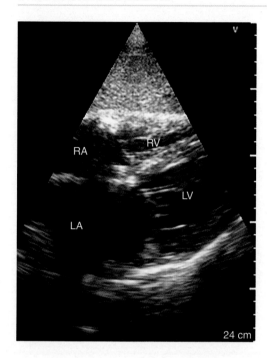

Fig. 6.10 Four-chamber view from the subcostal view showing the left ventricle (LV), right ventricle (RV), left atrium (LA), right atrium (RA), mitral valve, and tricuspid valve. Shown from top to bottom are the liver, RV inferior wall, RV cavity, inferior interventricular septum, LV cavity, and LV lateral wall.

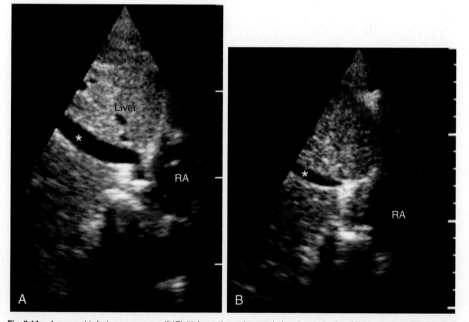

Fig. 6.11 A normal inferior vena cava (IVC) (*) from the subcostal view in expiration (A) inspiration (B). The IVC diameter 1 to 2 cm below the right atrium (RA) junction is less than 2.1 cm (A). There is greater than a 50% decrease in IVC diameter with inspiration (B) indicating a normal right atrial pressure.

Cardiovascular Case Studies Diagnosed With Handheld Echocardiography

CHAPTER 7

Case 1—A 70-Year-Old Man With Postoperative Atrial Fibrillation

History

- Cardiology consultation was obtained for a 70-year-old man for atrial fibrillation (AF) after a second knee arthroplasty surgery during current admission. Patient was on coumadin, and it had been restarted postoperatively.
- He had a history of AF perioperatively for knee arthroplasty 4 years ago.
- Patient had undergone mechanical mitral valve replacement 9 years ago for bioprosthetic mitral valve regurgitation (MR), which had initially been placed in the setting of severe MR as a result of mitral valve prolapse.
- An electrocardiogram (ECG) was performed (Fig. 7.1) and showed atrial flutter with a 4:1 block and a heart rate (HR) of 75 bpm.

Physical Examination

- Patient was stable and physical examination was unremarkable without cardiac murmurs. A handheld echocardiogram (HHE) was performed during cardiac consultation (Figs. 7.2, 7.3A-B, 7.4A-B, and 7.5A-B; Videos 7.1 and 7.2). HHE showed normal left ventricular (LV) and right ventricular (RV) systolic function and a normally functioning Carbomedics prosthetic mitral valve with normal disk motion and no pathologic MR. There was no pericardial effusion.

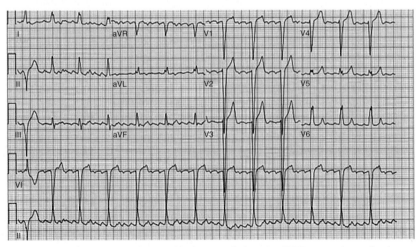

Fig. 7.1 ECG showed atrial flutter with a 4:1 block, a ventricular rate of 75 bpm, and occasional premature ventricular contraction.

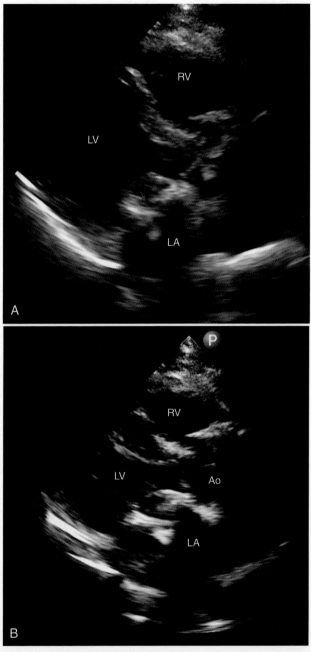

Fig. 7.2   Handheld echocardiogram parasternal long-axis view (PLAX) in diastole (A) and systole (B) showing normal left ventricle (LV) size and LV and RV systolic function based on change in cavity size. A mechanical valve is present in the mitral position (yellow arrows A and B). *Ao*, Aortic root; *LA*, left atrium; *RA*, right atrium; *RV*, right ventricle.

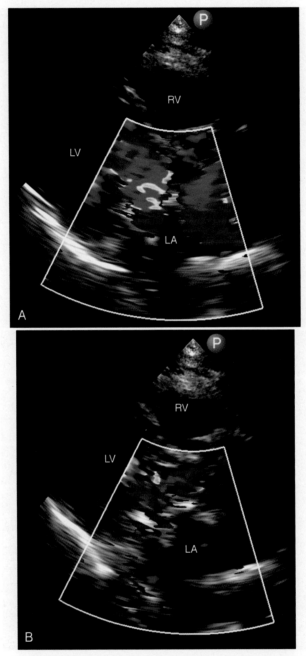

Fig. 7.3   HHE parasternal long-axis view (PLAX) color Doppler showing normal mitral diastolic inflow into the left ventricle (LV) without turbulence (A) and no blue flow into the left atrium (LA) in systole and normal homogenous forward flow into the aortic valve (B) indicating no mitral regurgitation and no aortic stenosis. *RV*, Right ventricle.

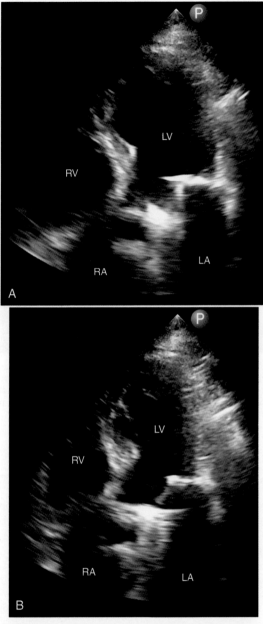

Fig. 7.4 HHE apical 5-chamber view in diastole (A) and systole (B) showing prosthetic mitral valve (red arrows A and B) and normal biventricular function. The mitral prosthesis inflow is directed toward LV outflow tract, not an uncommon occurrence because of surgical anatomy after two previous mitral valve surgeries. Also shown are significant biatrial enlargement and mild right ventricular enlargement based on a basal RV diameter of 43 mm (A). *LA*, Left atrium; *LV*, left ventricle; *RA*, right atrium; *RV*, right ventricle.

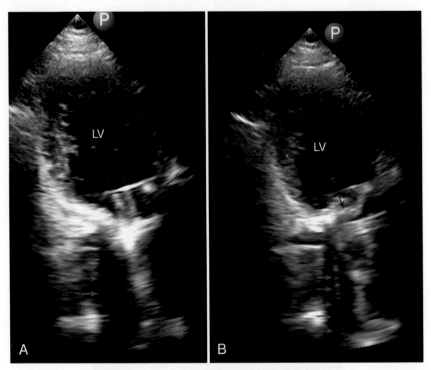

Fig. 7.5   HHE apical 2-chamber view in diastole (A) and systole (B) showing normal mitral prosthetic valve disk motion. Note parallel alignment of the mitral valve disks in the fully open position in diastole in (A) (red arrows) indicating a lack of pannus or thrombus obstructing disk motion. Normal closed prosthetic valve disks in systole are shown in (B) (red arrows). Shadowing from mitral prosthesis ring and reverberation from disk motion is shown in (A) (yellow arrows A and B). *LV*, Left ventricle.

Hospital Course

- Patient was given intravenous (IV) metoprolol, followed by oral metoprolol.
- He was discharged in atrial flutter with good rate control on metoprolol tartrate 25 mg twice daily and on coumadin for outpatient follow-up.
- No formal echocardiogram was obtained during this admission.

Final Diagnosis

Paroxysmal AF with normal ventricular and mechanical mitral valve function.

Utility of HHE in Patient Management

HHE helped assess cardiac function and mechanical mitral valve during AF and showed normal cardiac and valve function. This helped select pharmacologic management strategy. HHE ultrasound may be used to confirm normal mechanical valve function in a patient with no other clinical indication for mechanical valve dysfunction.

Teaching Point

HHE can help with assessment of global cardiac function during atrial flutter/fibrillation and help with determination of management strategy such as choice of atrioventricular nodal blocking agents, including negative inotropic agents such as diltiazem if the cardiac function is normal.

Case 2—Tight Wedding Ring on a 68-Year-Old Man With Dilated Cardiomyopathy and New Onset Atrial Fibrillation

History

- A 68-year-old man with a history of nonischemic cardiomyopathy with automatic implantable cardioverter defibrillator (AICD) implant developed fatigue and weight gain after a recent dental bone grafting procedure requiring pain control with nonsteroidal antiinflammatory agents
- He developed a 15-lb weight gain which partially responded to an increased dose of furosemide with loss of 9 lbs and presented to the emergency room with a 24-hour history of palpitations
- During an outpatient appointment for weight gain 5 days before presentation, a standard echocardiogram showed sinus rhythm, left ventricular ejection fraction (LVEF) of 31% (Figs. 7.6 and 7.7, Videos 7.3 and 7.4), moderate mitral regurgitation (Fig. 7.7, Video 7.4), and restrictive LV filling pattern (Figs. 7.8 and 7.9)
- An ECG performed during office visit had shown sinus rhythm.

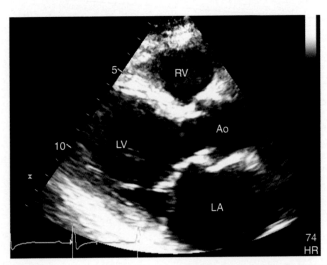

Fig. 7.6 Parasternal long-axis view by standard echocardiogram showing dilated left ventricle (LV) in end systole, left atrial enlargement, and posterior mitral leaflet prolapse (red arrow). *Ao,* Aorta; *LA,* left atrium; *RV,* right ventricle.

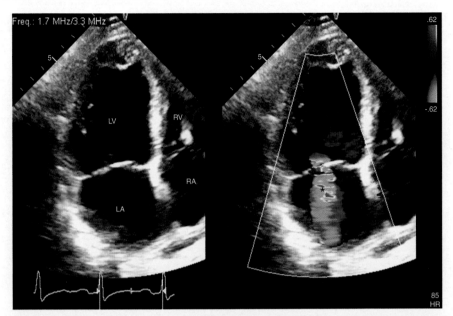

Fig. 7.7 Apical 4-chamber view by standard echocardiogram with the 2D image on the left and color Doppler across the mitral valve on the right showing left ventricle (LV) and left atrial (LA) enlargement, and moderate central mitral regurgitation by color Doppler (black asterisk). *RA,* Right atrium; *RV,* right ventricle.

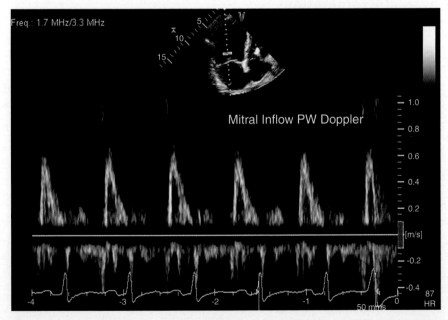

Fig. 7.8 Pulsed-wave (PW) Doppler mitral inflow by standard echocardiogram showing predominant E wave and insignificant A wave despite presence of sinus rhythm as a result of relative tachycardia (HR 83 bpm) and elevated level of left ventricle (LV) end-diastolic pressure.

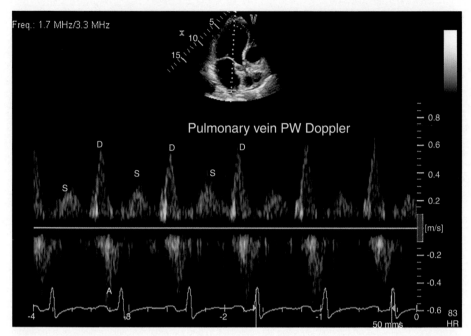

Fig. 7.9 Pulsed-wave (PW) Doppler of pulmonary vein showing restrictive pulmonary vein filling pattern (small S wave, tall D wave) and prominent atrial reversal (A wave) consistent with increased left atrial (LA) pressure (>15 mm Hg).

Physical Examination

- There was jugular venous distention and bilateral 1+ pitting ankle edema.

Laboratory Data and Diagnostics

- N-terminal-pro hormone B-type natriuretic peptide (NT-ProBNP) was 5107 pg/mL at presentation [3217 pg/mL 5 days ago (normal = 95 pg/mL)], serum creatinine was 1.2 mg/dL (normal).
- Increasing NT-ProBNP and weight gain indicated worsening heart failure in the patient.
- ECG was performed (Fig. 7.10) and the patient was found to be in new-onset atrial fibrillation (AF).

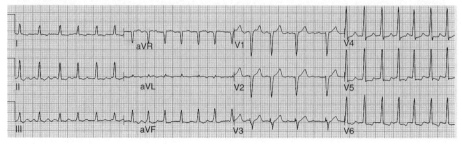

Fig. 7.10 12-Lead ECG at presentation showing atrial fibrillation with rapid ventricular response and ST/T wave changes in the lateral leads.

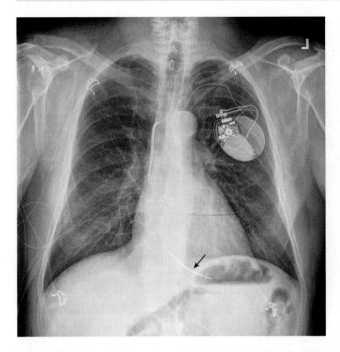

Fig. 7.11 Chest x-ray showing interstitial pulmonary congestion and defibrillator leads in right ventricle (red arrow).

- Chest x-ray (CXR) (Fig. 7.11) showed pulmonary venous congestion.
- Bedside handheld echocardiography (HHE) was performed during consultation and showed marked worsening of LV function compared with the recent standard echocardiogram in the parasternal long axis (Fig. 7.12, Video 7.5) and apical 4-chamber view (Fig. 7.13, Video 7.6). MR was moderate (Fig. 7.14).

Hospital Course

- The patient was started on apixaban 5 mg twice a day for anticoagulation and IV diuretics with a good diuretic response.
- Amiodarone infusion was started as a result of recent onset of AF of 24 hours. Over the next 12 hours, heart rates were still elevated in the 110s to 120s.
- As a result of persistent AF and congestive heart failure exacerbation, transesophageal echocardiogram (TEE)-guided cardioversion was planned.
- The patient was transported to the preoperative area to prepare for TEE cardioversion and was asked to remove his wedding ring by the nurse.
- Because of a mild, residual finger edema he had some difficulty removing the wedding ring, and he had to pull quite forcefully on his finger to remove the ring.
- During the maneuver, he converted to normal sinus rhythm.
- TEE was cancelled. Patient was transitioned to oral amiodarone 400 mg twice a day for 1 week for outpatient follow-up.

Final Diagnosis

- Acute exacerbation of congestive heart failure caused by new-onset AF and volume overload with underlying nonischemic dilated cardiomyopathy.

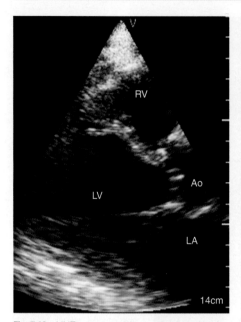

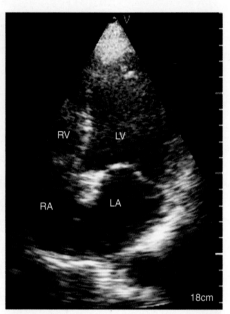

Fig. 7.12 HHE parasternal long-axis view showing an increase in left ventricle (LV) size than the standard echocardiogram performed before admission. *Ao,* Aorta; *LA,* left atrium; *RV,* right ventricle.

Fig. 7.13 Apical 4-chamber view with HHE showing increase in left ventricle (LV) size and worse LV function than standard echocardiogram shown earlier. *LA,* Left atrium; *RA,* right atrium; *RV,* right ventricle.

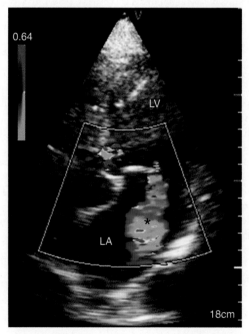

Fig. 7.14 HHE apical 4-chamber color Doppler view showing moderate mitral regurgitation (black asterisk). *LA,* Left atrium; *LV,* left ventricle.

Utility of HHE in Clinical Management

- HHE demonstrated marked worsening of cardiac function and mitral regurgitation.
- The physician avoided use of standard echocardiogram for repeat evaluation of cardiac function.

Teaching Point

- AF may result in the development of, or exacerbation of, congestive heart failure.
- Vagal maneuver has been shown to slow atrial flutter—and sometimes, AF—and convert AV node re-entry tachycardia.
- However, vagal maneuver does not generally convert AF to sinus rhythm; hence AF is treated with pharmacologic rate or rhythm control or with electrical cardioversion.
- The Valsalva maneuver is generally safe and well tolerated and can be performed before other vagal maneuvers or administration of medications, such as adenosine in patients with supraventricular tachyarrhythmia. It may occasionally convert sympathetically mediated AF, especially in a background of beta blockade and antiarrhythmics, to normal sinus rhythm.

Case 3—Resuscitated Cardiac Arrest After Coronary Artery Bypass Graft (CABG) Surgery and Mitral Valve Repair for Ischemic Mitral Regurgitation (MR)

History

- A 76-year-old man presented to the ED with altered level of consciousness after a successful resuscitation from cardiac arrest by a neighbor nurse.
- Past medical history was significant for prior myocardial infarction (MI), coronary artery bypass graft (CABG) and mitral valve repair surgery, atrial fibrillation, hypertension, dyslipidemia, ventricular tachycardia, and gastrointestinal bleed.
- Recent coronary angiogram done for ventricular tachycardia (VT) episodes had shown a patent single vein graft to the ramus intermedius and a normal left internal mammary artery (LIMA) graft to the distal left anterior descending (LAD) with occluded vein grafts to obtuse marginal (OM) 1 and 2 and vein graft to the right coronary artery (RCA).
- He underwent a biventricular upgrade of a dual-chamber implantable cardioverter defibrillator (ICD) performed 2 years before presentation.

Cardiac Workup

- ECG (Fig. 7.15) showed sinus rhythm with atrio-biventricular pacing. Chest x-ray (CXR), (Fig. 7.16) showed cardiomegaly, and cardiac and noncardiac pulmonary edema.
- ICD with pacemaker leads in RV and RA and a quadripolar LV lead in the coronary sinus branch.
- Chest CT scan (Fig. 7.17) confirmed pulmonary edema but also showed interstitial lung disease.
- Handheld echocardiography was performed and showed a normally functioning mitral annuloplasty ring without residual mitral regurgitation (MR), a dilated LV with reduced ejection fraction, an aneurysmal basal lateral segment with akinesis of basal and mid-inferolateral and mid-lateral segments along with a dyskinetic LV apex (Fig. 7.18, Video 7.7), and mildly elevated right atrial pressure by IVC evaluation (Fig. 7.19, Video 7.8).

Hospital Course

- Electrophysiology (EP) was consulted and ICD lead interrogation revealed two episodes of polymorphic VT in the setting of a recent reduction in amiodarone dose from 200 mg daily to 100 mg because of reduced diffusing lung capacity of oxygen (DLCO). There was a suspicion of border zone VT between infarcted and noninfarcted myocardium.

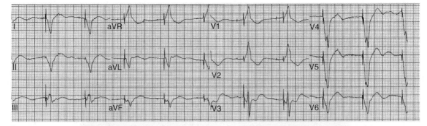

Fig. 7.15 ECG showing sinus rhythm with atrio-biventricular pacing.

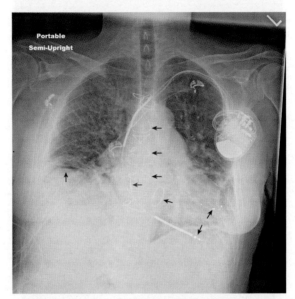

Fig. 7.16 Chest x-ray showing cardiomegaly with marked bilateral interstitial pulmonary edema, elevated right hemidiaphragm (light blue arrow), prior sternotomy wires (green arrows), pacemaker with implantable cardioverter defibrillator (ICD) lead (red arrow) in right ventricle (RV), right atrial (RA) lead (yellow arrow), and a quadripolar left ventricle (LV) lead (black arrow). A complete mitral annuloplasty ring (dark blue arrow) is also visualized.

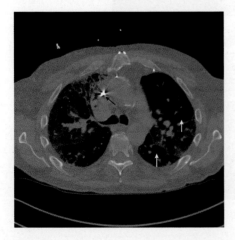

Fig. 7.17 CT scan shows pacemaker lead (black arrow). Increased opacities in the lung fields represent pulmonary edema and interstitial lung disease. Bullae (white arrows) are also shown.

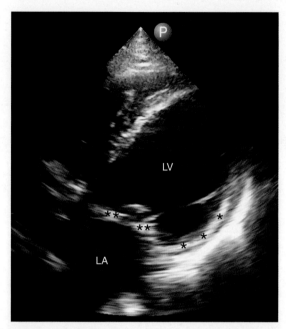

Fig. 7.18   Handheld echocardiographic subcostal 4-chamber view showing a mitral annuloplasty ring (double black asterisks), dilated left ventricle (LV) with thin and akinetic basal to mid-lateral wall (single black asterisks). *LA,* Left atrium.

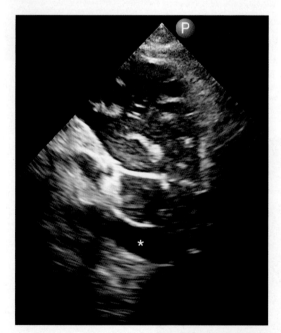

Fig. 7.19   HHE subcostal view showing dilated inferior vena cava (single white asterisk) indicating mild elevation of right atrial pressure.

- The origin of VT was felt to be in the border zone between aneurysmal and akinetic (subtended by occluded OM1 and OM2 vein grafts) and nonischemic myocardium.
- Patient was managed with increased amiodarone dose to 200 mg daily. Mexiletine 150 mg twice daily was added and heart failure regimen of beta blockers, ACE inhibitors, and spironolactone was up-titrated; and outpatient follow up was arranged.

Utility of HHE in Patient Management

- HHE showed dilated LV with markedly reduced LVEF.
- It also revealed the presence of a myocardial scar in the left circumflex (LCx) coronary artery territory (caused by two occluded vein grafts to OM1 and OM2).
- It showed a normally functioning mitral annuloplasty ring and mildly elevated right atrial pressure.
- Findings helped determine the potential etiology of polymorphic VT and appropriate antiarrhythmic and heart failure therapy.

Teaching Point: Ventricular Tachycardia in Coronary Artery Disease

- Monomorphic ventricular tachycardia in patients with prior MI is caused by re-entry within a scar.
- Polymorphic VT usually occurs at the border zone of ischemic and infarcted myocardium.
- The patient had the substrate for ischemia from occluded grafts and prior dense LCx territory infarct.
- Beta blockers and amiodarone are the main pharmacologic agents for symptomatic VT in CAD and low LVEF.
- Sotalol may be used in some patients.
- Mexiletine may be effective for short-term treatment for recurrent VT or VT storm in patients with CAD when amiodarone is ineffective or contraindicated.

CHAPTER 8

Case 1—A 72-Year-Old Man With Dysphagia, Dyspnea, and Ankle Edema

History

- A 78-year-old man presented with worsening dysphagia, dyspnea, and ankle edema.
- He had a history of coronary artery disease status post prior coronary artery stenting, congestive heart failure (CHF), ischemic cardiomyopathy requiring an implantable cardioverter defibrillator (ICD) and biventricular (Biv) pacemaker, hypertension, obstructive sleep apnea, and paroxysmal atrial fibrillation (AF).
- Laboratory values: N-terminal-pro hormone B-type natriuretic peptide (NT-proBNP): 8850 pg/mL (normal <325 pg/mL); creatinine clearance: 59 mL/min/m²; serum creatinine: 1.17 mg/dL (normal 0.5-1.2 mg/dL).
- Standard transthoracic echocardiogram (TTE) at admission showed marked left ventricular (LV) dysfunction with an ejection fraction of 24%, severe mitral regurgitation (MR), severe left atrial enlargement, and severe generalized LV hypokinesis.

Hospital Management

- For exacerbation of CHF and severely reduced LV function, furosemide continuous infusion was initiated that resulted in marked diuresis and resolution of dysphagia, dyspnea, and peripheral edema. Dysphagia was considered secondary to marked left atrial (LA) enlargement compressing the esophagus.
- ECG: on admission (Fig. 8.1) showed sinus rhythm; however, QRS morphology and width had changed compared to prior ECG.
- Anteroposterior (AP) chest x-ray (CXR) (Fig. 8.2) showed cardiomegaly, interstitial pulmonary edema, bilateral pleural effusions (left greater than right), and right atrial (RA), right ventricular (RV), and LV pacemaker leads in the appropriate location.
- To determine the burden of AF and adequacy of Biv pacing, pacemaker interrogation was performed, which demonstrated decreased LV lead capture with only 82% LV pacing and 90% RV pacing. There was 30% AF burden with ventricular response during AF of >120/min.
- LV lead amplitude was increased, which allowed good LV capture. Repeat ECG (Fig. 8.3) showed QRS morphology similar to patient's old ECG, although patient developed recurrent AF. Patient was on anticoagulation and beta blockers were continued as tolerated.
- Subsequent to initial diuresis and pacemaker programming, handheld endocardiography (HHE) was performed and showed slight reduction in LV size and slight improvement in left ventricular ejection fraction (LVEF) (Fig. 8.4A–B, Video 8.1), compared with the initial standard TTE as well as reduction in MR, which was now in the moderate range.

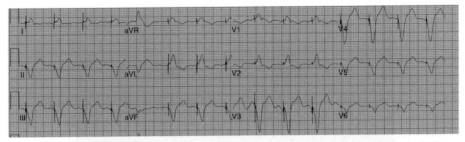

Fig. 8.1 ECG during current admission showing sinus rhythm with an A-sensed V-paced rhythm. QRS was wider with a change in QRS axis with reduced left ventricule (LV) capture compared with prior ECG. An isolated premature ventricular contraction (PVC) is also present.

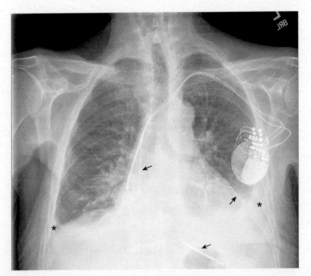

Fig. 8.2 Anteroposterior (AP) chest x-ray showing cardiomegaly, perihilar and basilar interstitial pulmonary edema, bilateral pleural effusions (black asterisks), left ventricule (LV) lead in the coronary sinus branch (black arrow), right atrial (red arrows), and right ventricular pacemaker/defibrillator lead (blue arrows).

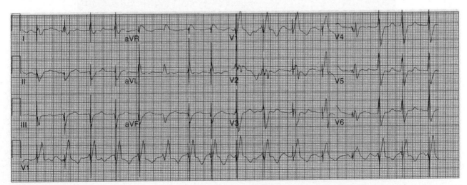

Fig. 8.3 The ECG was obtained after increasing the amplitude of the left ventricle (LV) lead to allow LV capture showing atrial fibrillation and reversal to the original QRS configuration as before admission.

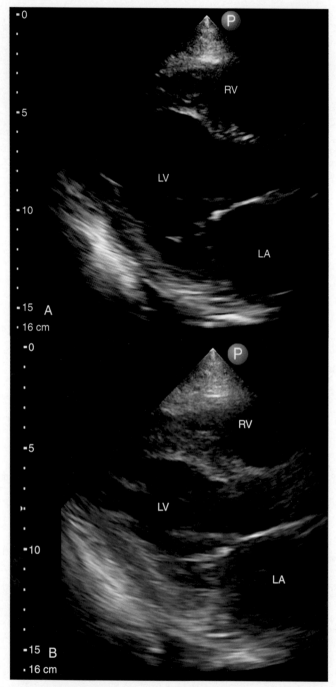

Fig. 8.4   HHE parasternal long-axis views showing (A) dilated left ventricle (LV), right ventricle (RV), and left atrium (LA) in end diastole and (B) dilated LV, RV, and LA in end systole and an improvement in left ventricular ejection fraction (LVEF) from baseline standard transthoracic echocardiogram (TTE).

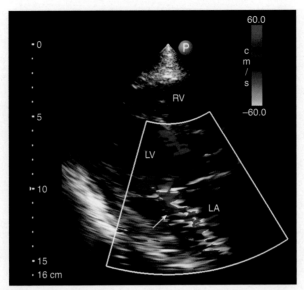

Fig. 8.5   HHE parasternal long-axis view showing moderate central jet of mitral regurgitation (white arrow). *LA,* Left atrium; *LV,* left ventricle; *RV,* right ventricle.

(Fig. 8.5). RV was moderately dilated and markedly hypokinetic (Fig. 8.6, Video 8.1) with moderate tricuspid regurgitation (TR). Inferior vena cava (IVC) and hepatic veins were dilated (Fig. 8.7, Video 8.2) and suggestive of persistent marked elevation of RA pressure. Large bilateral pleural effusions were also present on posterior lower chest imaging. Left lower chest imaging also showed cardiac image, although there was L pleural effusion as shown in Fig. 8.8.

Hospital Course

- As a result of persistent dyspnea and presence of significant bilateral pleural effusions on HHE, the patient underwent pleurocentesis over 48 hours with removal of 1000 and 600 mL fluid from the L and R sides respectively and a marked improvement in dyspnea.
- Patient became mobile on the floor.
- Subsequently the patient became hypotensive with increased O_2 requirements and was diagnosed with aspiration pneumonia.
- Inotropic support with dopamine and dobutamine infusion was initiated for worsening of CHF and renal function; however, hypotension remained unresponsive to inotropic support.
- Because of advanced irreversible cardiac dysfunction and after discussion with the family, palliative and comfort care was pursued and the patient died 7 days after admission.

Utility of HHE in Patient Management

- HHE may be helpful in hospital management of patients with CHF exacerbation with underlying ischemic cardiomyopathy.
  - HHE may allow follow-up assessment of RV size and function and right atrial pressure
  - HHE helped physicians titrate heart failure and diuretic therapy by assessment of volume status, LV size and function, and severity of MR and TR.
- HHE may help evaluate the size and location of pleural effusions and whether or not the patient would benefit from pleurocentesis.

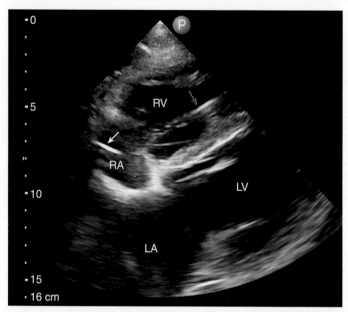

Fig. 8.6 HHE subcostal view showing enlargement of left and right heart chambers along with right ventricle (RV) (yellow arrow) and right atrial (RA) leads (white arrow). *LA,* Left atrium; *LV,* left ventricle.

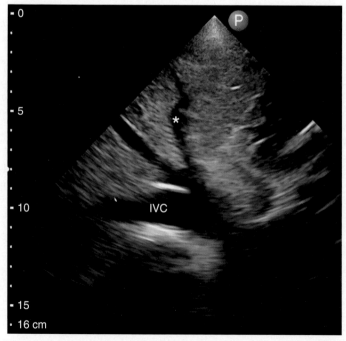

Fig. 8.7 HHE subcostal view showing dilated inferior vena cava (IVC) and hepatic vein (white asterisk).

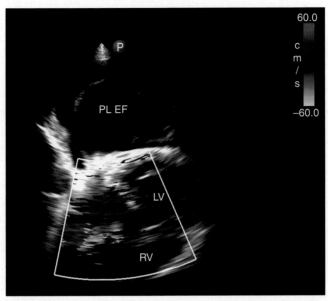

Fig. 8.8 Handheld echocardiographic image from the left flank showing left pleural effusion (PL EF). LV inferolateral wall is shown adjacent to the L pleural effusion. *LV,* Left ventricle; *RV,* right ventricle.

Final Diagnosis

Ischemic cardiomyopathy with heart failure exacerbation and nonresponse to cardiac resynchronization therapy (CRT).

Teaching Point

- In patients with prior Biv pacemaker implants who present with CHF, causes of nonresponse to Biv pacing should be sought.[1] These include presence of AF or supraventricular arrythmias, significant ventricular ectopy/arrhythmias, suboptimal atrioventricular delay programming, left atrial dysfunction, lead dislodgement, fracture or increased LV lead threshold leading to reduced LV pacing, presence of LV myocardial scar at the site of LV lead placement, significant valvular dysfunction, development of renal insufficiency, dietary or medication noncompliance, pneumonia, anemia, and RV failure.
- LV lead failure to capture allows continued RV pacing with detrimental effects on LV function.
- Attempts should be made to increase the percentage of Biv pacing by treating the underlying cause(s). In patients who are good candidates, LV lead replacement or repositioning may be required to improve Biv-pacing percentage. Very advanced cardiac dysfunction is often unresponsive to these measures.
- Referral for palliative care as opposed to advanced LV device support therapies should be performed based on age, other comorbidities, and goals of patient care.

References

1. Sieniewicz B, Gould J, Porter, Sidh BS, Teall T, Webb J, Carr-White G, Rinaldi CA. Understanding nonresponse to cardiac resynchronisation therapy: common problems and potential solutions. *Heart Failure Reviews.* 2019;24:41–54.

Case 2—A 78-Year-Old Man With Dysphagia and Known Coronary Artery Disease

History

- Cardiology was consulted to evaluate a 78-year-old Caucasian man before undergoing anesthesia for upper endoscopy and possible dilatation of esophageal stricture that had been dilated twice before.
- Patient had a history of left anterior descending (LAD) territory myocardial infarction (MI). An old nuclear scan had demonstrated infarct involving 15% of the myocardium subsequent to which the patient had undergone coronary artery bypass surgery. A recent evaluation had shown an LV ejection fraction of 51%.
- Patient had also presented with inferior ST-elevation MI 2 1/2 months before this consultation and underwent a drug-eluting stent placement in severely stenotic and thrombus-laden mid-right coronary artery. In addition, stenting of the 80% to 90% ostial circumflex coronary lesion and of a 50% left main lesion was also performed at the same time.
- Patient had now presented with recurrent dysphagia and inability to swallow fluids.

ECG

ECG (Fig. 8.9) showed QS complexes in leads V2 and V3 and Q waves in leads V4-V6 indicative of a prior anterior/apical transmural infarct.

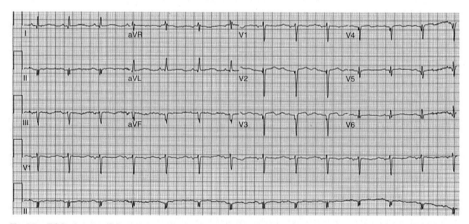

Fig. 8.9   ECG showing QS complexes in the anterior precordial leads V2-V4 with mild ST elevation. An left ventricle (LV) apical aneurysm can be diagnosed on ECG when there is persistent ST segment elevation occurring for 6 weeks and often associated with well-formed Q waves or with QS complexes in the anterior precordial leads after a known transmural mayocardial infarction (MI). Pathologic Q waves in leads II, AVF, V5, and V6 is suggestive of an old right coronary artery (RCA) territory MI with posterolateral extension.

Handheld Echocardiography

- Bedside echocardiogram was performed, which revealed a left ventricular apical aneurysm from an old LAD MI without obvious apical thrombus, endocardial brightness, and hypoakinesis of mid-inferolateral wall. An overall preserved left ventricular ejection fraction in the parasternal long axis (Fig. 8.10, Video 8.3), the apical 4-chamber view (not shown), and mild-to-moderate central mitral regurgitation (Fig. 8.11) are present.
- A standard echocardiogram confirmed the findings of HHE. As a result of apical foreshortening, contrast enhancement was performed and did not show LV apical thrombus.

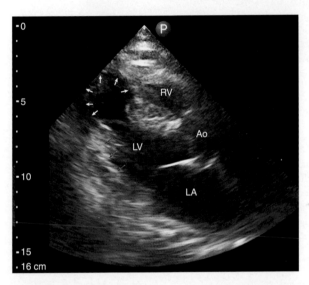

Fig. 8.10 Parasternal long-axis view showing left ventricle (LV) apical aneurysm involving distal interventricular septum, LV apex, and distal inferolateral wall (*white arrows*). Endocardial brightness of the mid inferolateral wall is present because of an old right coronary artery (RCA) myocardial infarction (MI) (*yellow arrows*). Global left ventricular ejection fraction (LVEF) was mildly reduced and LV size appears normal.

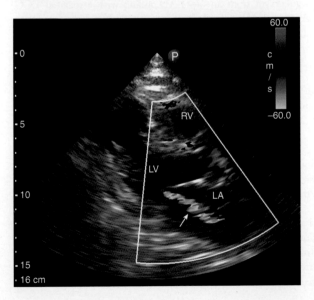

Fig. 8.11 Parasternal long-axis view with color Doppler showing mild-to-moderate mitral regurgitation (white arrow).

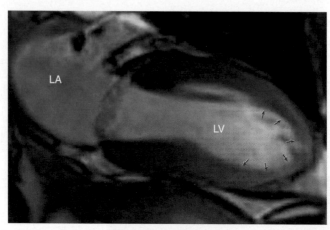

Fig. 8.12 Cardiac MRI showing aneurysmal left ventricle (LV) apex (yellow arrows) in the 2-chamber view and with no LV thrombus. *LA,* Left atrium.

Hospital Course

- Cardiology recommended that the patient undergoes endoscopy without stopping clopidogrel bisulfate given his recent multivessel coronary stent intervention.
- Cardiac MRI was performed and confirmed apical aneurysm with increased gadolinium enhancement suggestive of an apical myocardial scar (Fig. 8.12).
- A subsequent nuclear scintigraphy scan was performed and showed an irreversible apical perfusion defect.

Final Diagnosis

The diagnosis was an LV apical aneurysm from an old LAD infarct with associated ECG changes and an old dominant RCA territory MI without significant mitral regurgitation and with preserved LV function.

Utility of HHE in Clinical Management

- It demonstrated a preserved LV systolic function with an old apical aneurysm from a prior LAD territory infarct, no significant valvular dysfunction, and no mobile LV apical thrombus.

Teaching Point

- A true LV aneurysm is defined as a well delineated, thin, scarred, or fibrotic wall, devoid of muscle or containing necrotic muscle, that is a result of a healed transmural MI. The involved wall segment is either akinetic (without movement) or dyskinetic (with paradoxical outward systolic motion).
- Aneurysms of the apex and anterior wall are more than four times as common as those of the inferior or inferoposterior walls.
- The incidence of LV apical true aneurysms has decreased from to 30% to 35% in patients with Q wave MI to about 8% to 15% because of rapid revascularization of infarct-related arteries by thrombolysis or primary percutaneous coronary intervention (PCI) in patients with acute MI.

- The presence and severity of ischemic MR should be evaluated in patients with a prior RCA or left circumflex (LCx) territory infarct particularly involving basal-to-mid segments and results from infarct remodeling at the site of posterior papillary muscle insertion, papillary muscle infarction and fibrosis, and chordal shortening.

True LV Aneurysm

- LV aneurysm is a frequent complication of acute MI that can lead to death or serious morbidity.
- LV apical aneurysms from LAD territory MI are more common than inferior or inferolateral wall aneurysms.
- Other causes of LV aneurysms include apical hypertrophic cardiomyopathy and Chagas disease.
- The aneurysm may be asymptomatic or present as heart failure, sustained ventricular tachyarrhythmias, or arterial embolism caused by development of a thrombus in the aneurysm.

Multimodality Imaging for LV Apical Aneurysm

- Two-dimensional transthoracic echocardiography is the first imaging study obtained in most patients. Contrast-enhanced TTE has a sensitivity and specificity of 64% and 95% to 98% respectively in the detection of LV thrombi.
- Cardiac computerized tomographic angiography has become the standard imaging test and can confirm the diagnosis in patients in whom two-dimensional echocardiography is not diagnostic.
- Radionuclide ventriculography or contrast ventriculography at the time of cardiac catheterization are alternatives.
- Three-dimensional echocardiography and magnetic resonance imaging are newer modalities that are increasingly used for diagnosis of LV aneurysms, for evaluation of the presence of thrombi, and for the assessment of myocardial viability by gadolinium enhancement.

CHAPTER 9

Case 1—A 75-Year-Old Woman With Known Advanced Cardiomyopathy Presents to the Emergency Department With Recurrent Dyspnea

History

A 75-year-old woman presented to the emergency department with increasing weight gain and shortness of breath. She was known to have nonischemic cardiomyopathy with a very poor ejection fraction of 14% and was being evaluated by palliative care. She took extra doses of the diuretic bumetanide (Bumex) with increased diuresis but came to the emergency room because of persistent exertional dyspnea.

Physical Examination

Jugular venous pressure was elevated to 10 cm H_2O. Cardiac examination revealed a displaced apical impulse in the anterior axillary line in the sixth intercostal space, an S3 gallop, and a 4/6 soft holosystolic apical murmur.

Laboratory Data

Hemoglobin, Hb: 13.3 g/dL; creatinine: 0.9 mg/dL; Troponin I, TnI: 25 ng/dL (normal <0.40 ng/mL); N-terminal proB-type natriuretic peptide, NT-proBNP: 2146 pg/mL (normal <450 pg/mL).

ECG: Showed sinus rhythm with first degree atrioventricular (AV) block, poor R wave progression in leads V1-V3, and voltage criteria for left ventricular hypertrophy (Fig. 9.1).

Chest X-ray, CXR: Showed cardiomegaly, bilateral pulmonary congestion, pacemaker/implantable cardioverter defibrillator (ICD) with leads in the right atrium (RA) and the right ventricle (RV), and no pleural effusions (Fig. 9.2).

HHE Findings in the Emergency Department

There was marked left ventricular enlargement with severe global hypokinesis and left ventricular (LV) dysfunction in the parasternal long axis (Figs. 9.3A–B, Video 9.1) and apical 4-chamber view (Figs. 9.4A–B) with an estimated left ventricular ejection fraction (LVEF) of 10% to 15%, severe functional mitral regurgitation caused by poor mitral leaflet coaptation with leaflet tenting (Fig. 9.5) causing low leaflet coaptation >1 cm below mitral annular plane (Fig. 9.3B), and moderately dilated inferior vena cava (IVC) (Fig. 9.6) with less than 50% inspiratory collapse suggestive of a right atrial (RA) pressure of 15 mm Hg.

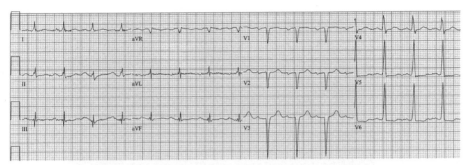

Fig. 9.1 ECG Showing Sinus Rhythm With First Degree AV Block, Poor R Wave Progression in Leads V1-V3, and Minor Voltage Criteria of Left Ventricular Hypertrophy. There was no RV pacing.

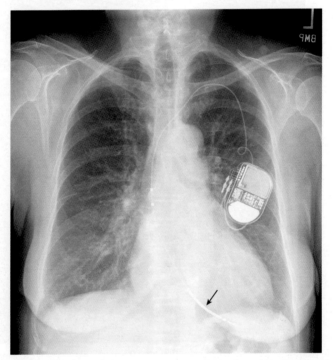

Fig. 9.2 CXR Showing Cardiomegaly With Left Subclavian Defibrillator Wire in Right Ventricle (Black Arrow) and Bilateral Pulmonary Venous Congestion.

Clinical Course

Clinical findings were consistent with exacerbation of congestive heart failure. Patient was given intravenous (IV) bumetanide 1 mg in the emergency room. This resulted in good diuresis; O_2 saturation improved from 90% upon arrival to 95% after diuresis. Patient walked in the hallway and was able to maintain O_2 saturation in the 93% range. She was discharged home with an increased dose of bumetanide from 2 mg twice a day to 3 mg twice a day with cardiology outpatient follow-up.

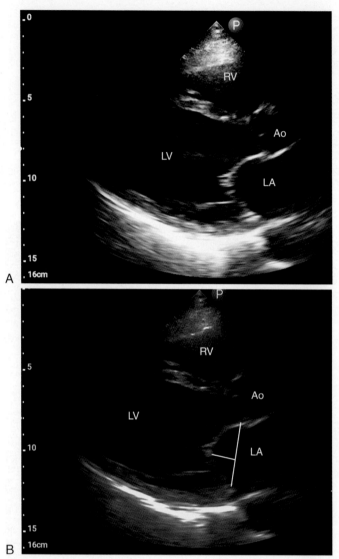

Fig. 9.3   (A) HHE parasternal long-axis view showing severe LV enlargement. There is moderate enlargement of RV outflow tract. (B) HHE parasternal long-axis view in end systole showing severe LV enlargement and global LV systolic dysfunction. There is moderate enlargement and moderate-to-severe dysfunction of the RV outflow tract. There is mitral leaflet tenting (measured as vertical distance of the mitral leaflet coaptation to the mitral annular plane and malcoaptation [red arrow]). *Ao,* Aortic root; *LA,* left atrium; *LV,* left ventricle; *RV,* right ventricle.

Utility of HHE in Clinical Management

HHE helped confirm clinical findings of heart failure exacerbation. It confirmed no new findings (such as pericardial effusion, LV thrombus, worsening of RV size or function) to explain heart failure exacerbation. It also helped determine acute management strategy and discharge from the emergency department.

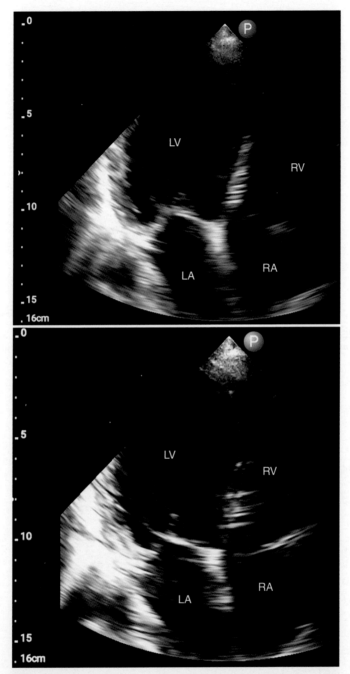

Fig. 9.4 (A) HHE apical 4-chamber view (LV on the left side) in end diastole showing LV and RV enlargement. (B) HHE apical 4-chamber view (LV on the left side) in end systole showing 4-chamber enlargement and markedly reduced LV systolic function. *LA,* Left atrium; *LV,* left ventricle; *RA,* right atrium; *RV,* right ventricle.

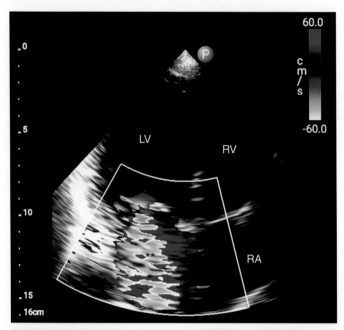

Fig. 9.5   HHE Apical 4-Chamber View (LV on the Left Side) Showing Severe Central Jet of Mitral Regurgitation (Double Black Asterisks). *LA*, Left atrium; *LV*, left ventricle; *RA*, right atrium; *RV*, right ventricle.

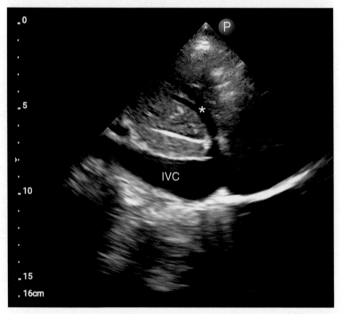

Fig. 9.6   HHE Subcostal View Showing Dilated Inferior Vena Cava (IVC) and Hepatic Vein (White Asterisk).

Final Diagnosis

Advanced nonischemic cardiomyopathy and severe functional mitral regurgitation.

Teaching Point

HHE may be used to characterize heart failure exacerbation and prevent hospital readmissions in select patients. The total cost of HF in the US for 2012 was $30.7 billion.[1] The median risk-standardized 30-day readmission rate for heart failure was 23.0% from 2009 to 2012.[2]

CHF exacerbations as well as repeat hospital admissions may be avoidable if appropriate triaging can be performed in patients' homes or in the ED. Although majority of heart failure readmissions are caused by noncardiovascular causes, among patients with readmissions secondary to heart failure exacerbation, majority are caused by congestion and may be recognizable by technologies such as HHE in outpatient clinics or in emergency rooms. A study by Chamberlain RS et al.[2] found the following criteria as risk factors for heart failure readmissions: age <65 years, male gender, first income quartile, African American race, race other than African American or Caucasian, Medicare, Medicaid, self-pay/no insurance, drug abuse, renal failure, chronic pulmonary disorder, diabetes, depression, and fluid and electrolyte disorders.

References

1. Mozaffarian D, Banjamin EJ, Go AS, et al. Heart disease and stroke statistics—2015 update: a report from the American Heart Association. *Circulation*. 2014;129:29-323.
2. Chamberlain RS, Sond J, Mahendraraj K, et al. Determining 30-day readmission risk for heart failure patients: The readmission after heart failure scale. *Int J Gen Med*. 2018;11:127-141.

Case 2—78-Year-Old Man With Lower Extremity Edema, Dyspnea, and Weight Gain During a Long Cruise

History

A 78-year-old Caucasian man presented with lower extremity edema, dyspnea, and weight gain. Symptoms developed during a recent prolonged cruise that lasted several weeks and did not respond to an increasing diuretic dosage of furosemide from 20 to 40 mg twice daily in addition to metolazone 2.5 mg once daily. Past medical history was significant for nonischemic dilated cardiomyopathy with left ventricular ejection fraction (LVEF) of 26% on an echocardiogram four months ago and a prior history of an implantable cardioverter defibrillator (ICD) implant. Coronary angiogram performed two months ago had shown normal coronary arteries. He also has a history of multiple myeloma not having achieved remission.

The patient had WHO type IV pulmonary artery hypertension from recurrent pulmonary thromboembolic disease and was on the anticoagulant, coumadin, and a pulmonary vasodilator, Riociguat.

Physical Examination

The patient was dyspneic during conversation and had a four-pillow orthopnea. Pulse was irregular. BP was 104/70 mm Hg. There was jugular venous distension and bilateral 2+ pitting edema up to the knees.

Electrocardiogram

Twelve-lead ECG showed atrial flutter with a ventricular rate of nearly 100 bpm (Fig. 9.7), which was new from his prior ECG.

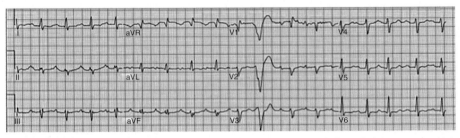

Fig. 9.7 Electrocardiogram upon admission showed atrial flutter with controlled ventricular response, which was new compared with sinus rhythm before.

Hospital Course

Intravenous diuretics were initiated immediately after admission. However, there was no significant response to a total IV furosemide dose of 160 mg overnight.

Implantable Cardioverter Defibrillator (ICD) Interrogation

ICD interrogation revealed a 7% right ventricular pacing and persistent atrial flutter for the last month and a half.

HHE Findings

Handheld echocardiogram (HHE) was performed during morning rounds. There was moderate-to-severe right ventricular enlargement (Figs. 9.8-9.11) and dysfunction (Videos 9.2 and 9.3), which was new from his past standard echocardiogram 2 months ago. There was mid-interventricular septal flattening (Figs. 9.8 and 9.11, Videos 9.2 and 9.3) suggestive of marked RV dysfunction and/or pulmonary hypertension. There was mild tricuspid regurgitation.

Left ventricular ejection fraction was estimated at 25% and RA pressure was estimated at 15 mm Hg from IVC evaluation. Subsequent standard echocardiogram confirmed LV systolic dysfunction (Fig. 9.12A-B), a RV-RA gradient of 36 mm Hg (Fig 13A), and marked reduction in RV stroke volume as measured by RV ejection velocity (Fig. 13B).

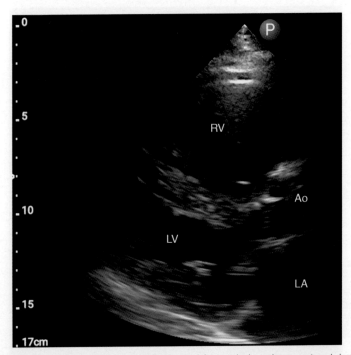

Fig. 9.8 HHE parasternal long-axis view showing severe right ventricular enlargement and dysfunction and interventricular septum (red arrow) flattening (red arrow) from RV dysfunction and volume and pressure overload (red arrow). *Ao,* Aortic root; *LA,* left atrium; *LV,* left ventricle; *RV,* right ventricle.

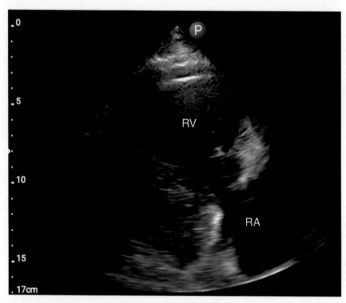

Fig. 9.9   HHE right ventricular inflow view showing severe RV and RA enlargement. *RA*, Right atrium; *RV*, right ventricle.

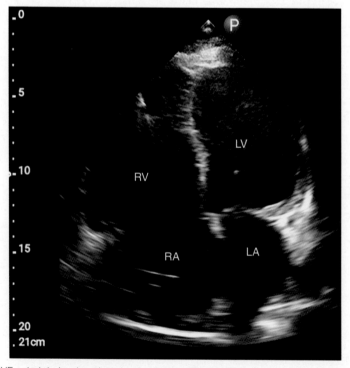

Fig. 9.10   HHE apical 4-chamber view showing marked RV and RA enlargement. *LA*, Left atrium; *LV*, left ventricle; *RA*, right atrium; *RV*, right ventricle.

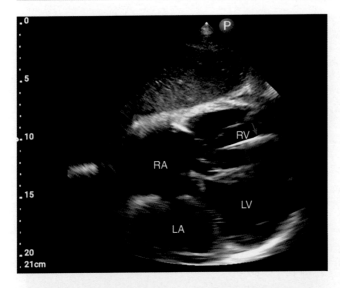

Fig. 9.11 HHE Subcostal View Showing Marked RV and RA Enlargement, Interventricular Septum (IVS) Flattening (Red Arrow), and ICD Lead in RV (Yellow Arrow). *LA*, Left atrium; *LV*, left ventricle; *RA*, right atrium; *RV*, right ventricle.

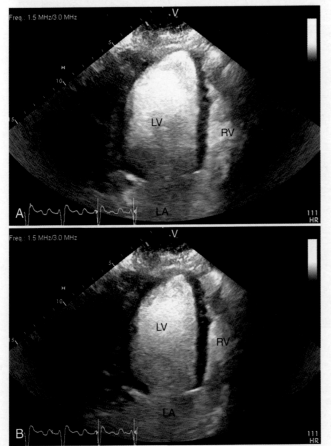

Fig. 9.12 (A) Microbubble-enhanced 4-chamber view in end diastole by standard echocardiogram showing LV enlargement. (B) Microbubble-enhanced 4-chamber view in end systole by standard echocardiogram showing LV systolic dysfunction. *LA*, Left atrium; *LV*, left ventricle; *RV*, right ventricle.

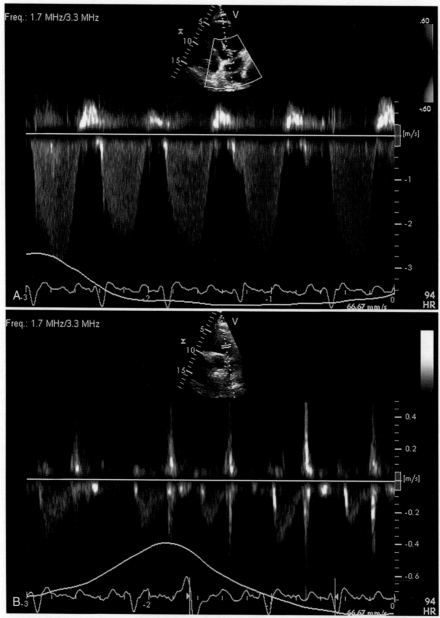

Fig. 9.13 (A) Continuous-wave doppler obtained with a standard echocardiogram showing Increased right ventricle–right atrium (RV-RA) gradient. Note atrial flutter on ECG. (B) Right ventricular outflow tract (RVOT) pulsed Doppler obtained with a standard echocardiogram showing markedly reduced RV outflow tract velocity and its time integral (RVOT VTI) consistent with markedly reduced RV systolic function. Beat-to-beat variability is caused by atrial flutter and respiratory variation as shown by respirogram superimposed on the ECG. Pulmonary vascular resistance can be estimated by echocardiogram using the formula: RV peak velocity/RVOT VTI × 10 + 0.6 (5.6 wood units in this case). RV myocardial index is calculated as TR velocity duration − RV ejection time/RV ejection time. Normal RV myocardial performance index (RV MPI) is 0.43. In this patient RV MPI was 0.8.

Initial Hospital Course

Bolus doses of diuretics were changed to infusion of furosemide at 10 mg/h with improvement in diuretic response.

On account of the findings and history of type IV pulmonary HTN, patient was referred for a right heart catheterization to determine severity of pulmonary artery pressure and pulmonary vascular resistance.

Right Heart Catheterization

RA pressure 11 mm Hg
PAP 44/22 mm Hg
Pulmonary vascular resistance 5.4 wood units
Pulmonary capillary wedge pressure 10 mm Hg
Transpulmonary gradient 20 mm Hg
Cardiac index 1.72 L/min/m^2

Subsequent Course

- A diagnosis of right heart failure with a mildly increased pulmonary artery pressure was made. Diuretics were held. Patient was started on a dobutamine drip at 3 μg/kg/min because of subsequent hypotension (70/50 mm Hg) without significant improvement.
- To increase cardiac output restoration of atrial function and conversion to sinus rhythm was considered important.
- Despite DNR (Do Not Resuscitate) status, a long discussion was held with the patient regarding benefits vs risk of sedation for a transesophageal echocardiography (TEE)-guided cardioversion and possible risks of intubation to exclude LA appendage thrombus (due to inadequate compliance with coumadin during the cruise). Patient agreed to proceed with temporary removal of DNR and DNI (Do Not Intubate) status.
- Direct current (DC) cardioversion was performed successfully on one attempt with 200 joules biphasic current after no thrombus was found on TEE.
- Subsequent to cardioversion the patient's blood pressure improved and he was able to tolerate heart failure medications.
- Patient was discharged and was alive at 9-month follow-up.

Utility of HHE in Clinical Management

HHE helped determine that the cause of heart failure was mostly related to right ventricular dilation and dysfunction in the setting of new-onset atrial flutter and dietary indiscretion during the cruise.

Final Diagnosis

Acute right heart failure with new-onset atrial flutter in the setting of advanced nonischemic dilated cardiomyopathy and type IV pulmonary hypertension.

Teaching Point

RIGHT VENTRICULAR DYSFUNCTION AND ECHOCARDIOGRAPHIC ASSESSMENT

The RV is able to withstand volume overload much better than pressure overload. RV dilation can maintain RV cardiac output for several years because of Starling's law in response to volume overload. However, RV cannot handle pressure overload in the same way as volume overload. If RV contractile response to pressure overload caused by left heart failure or primary lung or pulmonary vascular pathology (such as pulmonary embolism) fails, it causes acute RV dilation and dysfunction. This RV failure manifests as hypotension and cardiogenic shock.

Some of the mechanisms of right heart failure after left heart failure include: the same pathology affecting both ventricles, such as ischemia, myocarditis or cardiomyopathy, pulmonary venous hypertension caused by left heart failure, reduced RV coronary perfusion secondary to severely reduced LV cardiac output, and impaired RV filling caused by severe LV dilation and pericardial constraint.

Bedside echocardiogram allows rapid assessment of RV size and function and interventricular septum (IVS) shift. In the apical 4-chamber view, basal RV should be 1/3 the size of basal LV. An RV/LV basal diameter ratio of more than 1 can be useful in determining significant RV enlargement. Loss of LV sphericity resulting in a D-shaped LV is indicative of advanced RV volume or pressure overload. Flattening of the septum occurs in diastole in volume overload, in systole in pressure overload, and in both systole and diastole in advanced pulmonary hypertension.

Symptoms of right heart failure are mainly caused by systemic venous congestion and/or low cardiac output. These include exertional dyspnea, fatigue, dizziness, ankle swelling, epigastric fullness, and right upper abdominal discomfort or pain.

Diuretics to reduce RV preload and conversion to sinus rhythm should be performed when exacerbation of heart failure is precipitated by volume overload and new-onset atrial fibrillation (AF)/atrial flutter.

WORLD HEALTH ORGANIZATION CLASSIFICATION OF PULMONARY ARTERIAL HYPERTENSION

Group I: Idiopathic, Familial, PAH associated with other systemic diseases

Group II: Secondary to left heart disease (valvular heart disease, systolic LV dysfunction, diastolic LV dysfunction)

Group III: Associated with lung disease or hypoxemia (chronic obstructive pulmonary disease, interstitial lung disease, obstructive sleep apnea, chronic hypoxemia)

Group IV: Chronic thromboembolic disease

Group V: Miscellaneous (Sarcoidosis, mediastinitis)

Case 3—A 53-Year-Old Female With New Onset Heart Failure

A 53-year-old Caucasian woman presented with increasing lower extremity edema, New York Heart Association (NYHA) class III. There was jugular venous distention to the angle of the jaw at a 45% supine angle. There was 2+ pitting edema up to the knees. There were no murmurs.

ECG: Showed sinus rhythm with low voltage in the limb leads and infarct patterns in the inferior and anteroseptal leads (Fig. 9.14).

HHE was performed during office consultation and showed markedly increased LV wall thickness in a diffuse pattern in the parasternal long-axis view (Fig. 9.15 and Video 9.4), short-axis view (Fig. 9.16 and Video 9.5), and LV focused apical 4-chamber view (Fig. 9.17). Diffuse thickening of RV walls was seen in the RV-focused apical view (Fig. 9.18). There was small circumferential pericardial effusion seen in all these views. Posterior left lower chest imaging also showed pleural effusion and pericardial effusion (Fig. 9.19). IVC was markedly dilated with reduced inspiratory collapse (Figs. 9.20A-B, Video 9.6) suggestive of RA pressure between 15 mm Hg and 20 mm Hg.

Cardiac amyloidosis was suspected. Strain imaging was performed on the standard ultrasound (US) machine and showed apical preservation of strain and a global LV longitudinal strain (Fig. 9.21).

Laboratory Data

N-terminal proB-type natriuretic peptide, NT-proBNP: 3964 pg/mL (normal <450 pg/mL); Troponin T: 0.21 ng/mL (normal <0.01 ng/mL); IgA lambda monoclonal gammopathy, IgA level 1252 (normal 0.8 g/L-3 g/L).

Bone marrow biopsy was performed and showed 10% plasma cells. She was started on chemotherapy with Cyclophosphamide-Bortezomib-Dexamethasone (CyBorD) along with furosemide 40 mg twice a day and metolazone initially at 5 mg per day; and then, on an as-needed basis.

At 3-month follow-up, her NYHA functional class had improved to class II, Troponin T level was 0.02 ng/mL, and NT-proBNP level had decreased to 1542 pg/mL. Patient underwent successful autologous stem cell transplantation 4 months later. NT-proBNP at follow-up 5 months after stem cell transplant was 1317 pg/mL. An HHE showed regression of LV wall thickness (Fig. 9.22 and Video 9.7) and reduction in right atrial pressure (Fig. 9.23 and Video 9.8).

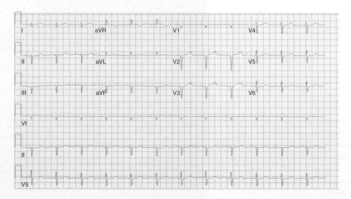

Fig. 9.14 Twelve-Lead ECG Showing Low Voltage and Pseudoinfarct Pattern in the Inferior and Anteroseptal Leads.

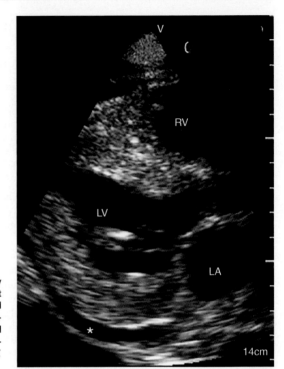

Fig. 9.15 Parasternal Long-Axis View by HHE Showing Diffuse Increase in Left Ventricular Wall Thickness With Ground Glass Appearance, Small LV End-Systolic Cavity, and a Small Circumferential Pericardial Effusion (Single White Asterisk). *LA,* Left atrium; *LV,* left ventricle; *RV,* right ventricle.

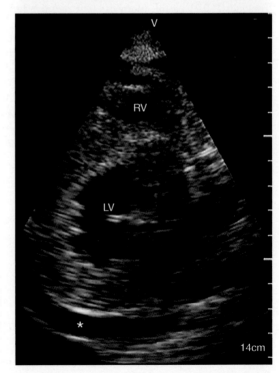

Fig. 9.16 Parasternal Short-Axis View Near Mid Ventricle by HHE Showing Diffuse Increase in Left Ventricular Wall Thickness With Ground Glass Appearance, Small LV End-Systolic Cavity, and A Small Circumferential Pericardial Effusion (Single White Asterisk). *LV,* Left ventricle; *RV,* right ventricle.

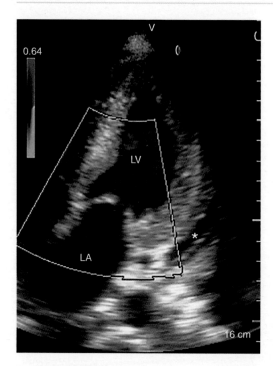

Fig. 9.17 Off-Axis Apical 4-Chamber View by HHE Showing Diffuse Increase in Ventricular Wall Thickness With Ground Glass Appearance, Small LV End-Diastole Cavity, and a Small Circumferential Pericardial Effusion (Single White Asterisk). *LA;* Left atrium; *LV,* left ventricle.

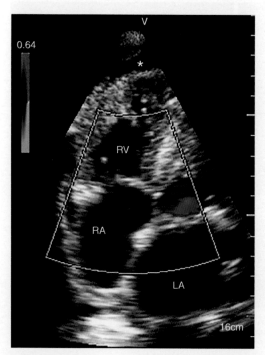

Fig. 9.18 Right Ventricular-Focused Apical 4-Chamber View by HHE Showing Diffuse Increase in RV Wall Thickness and a Small Circumferential Pericardial Effusion (Single White Asterisk). *LA,* Left atrium; *RA,* right atrium; *RV,* right ventricle.

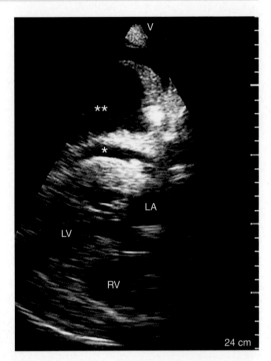

Fig. 9.19 Left Posterior Transthoracic Imaging With HHE Showing a Left Pleural Effusion (double white asterisks), a Small Circumferential Pericardial Effusion (single white asterisk), and Three Cardiac Chambers—the Left Atrium (LA), Left Ventricle (LV), and Right Ventricle (RV).

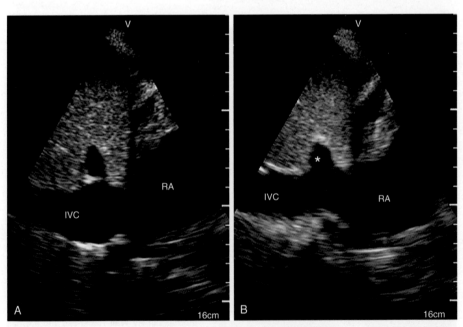

Fig. 9.20 (A) Subcostal imaging with HHE showing a moderately dilated IVC and hepatic vein (single white asterisk) during end expiration. (B) Subcostal imaging with HHE showing a <50% reduction in IVC diameter with a sniff. *IVC,* Inferrior vena cava; *RA,* right atrium.

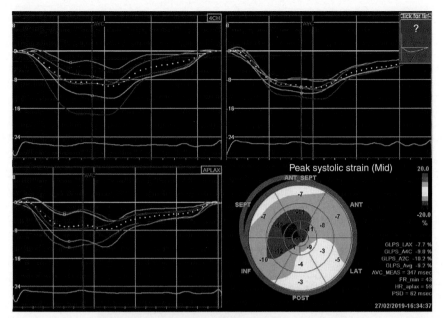

Fig. 9.21 Speckle-Tracking Longitudinal LV Strain Maps in Apical 3, 2 and Chamber Views in the Top Left, Top Right, and Bottom Left Panels, Respectively Showing Reduced Longitudinal Strain in All Segments. Bottom right panel is the bull's eye plot showing marked reduction in strain in all segments (pink and pale pink segments) with some preservation in the apical and periapical segments (red segments).

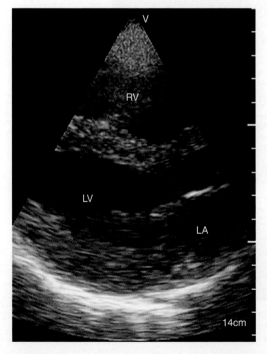

Fig. 9.22 Parasternal Long-Axis View by HHE 5 Months After Stem Cell Transplant Showing Marked Decrease in V Wall Thickness and No Pericardial Effusion. *LA*, Left atrium; *LV*, left ventricle; *RV*, right ventricle.

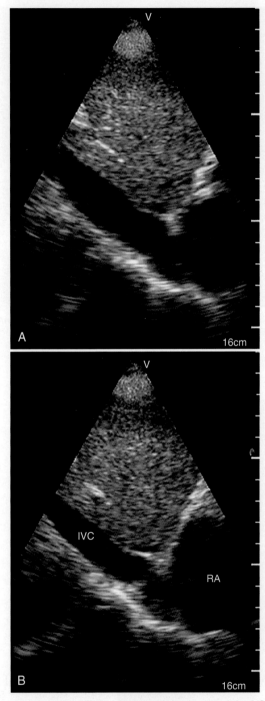

Fig. 9.23   (A) Subcostal imaging with HHE showing a reduction in size of the IVC during end expiration 5 months after stem cell transplant. (B) Subcostal imaging with HHE showing a 50% reduction in IVC diameter with a sniff. *IVC,* Inferior vena cava; *RA,* right atrium.

Teaching Point

Suspect infiltrative cardiomyopathy in a patient with low ECG voltage in the presence of marked increase in unexplained LV wall thickness or ECG LV thickness mismatch, diastolic dysfunction, ECG pseudoinfarct pattern, pericardial effusion, and increase in LV and RV filling pressures causing restrictive cardiomyopathy.

Role of HHE in Clinical Management

HHE allowed bedside diagnosis with subsequent confirmation by speckle tracking strain imaging and subsequent laboratory and biopsy data. Amyloidosis is a systemic disease characterized by extracellular deposition of amyloid protein into various organs. Cardiac infiltration of these misfolded proteins results in cardiac amyloidosis (CA). Amyloid light-chain (AL) cardiac amyloidosis is the most common type of infiltrative cardiomyopathy and is caused by bone marrow plasma cell dyscrasia causing an overproduction of immunoglobulin light chains. Transthyretin or ATTR amyloidosis includes a senile form (now reported to be present in as many as 16% of elderly patients undergoing Transcatheter Aortic Valve Replacement [TAVR]). The hereditary or familial type of TTR amyloid is more uncommon. AL amyloid has very poor survival measured in months, and TTR amyloidosis has survival measured in years.

AL amyloid is treated with chemotherapy and stem cell transplant. Liver transplant is used for the familial type of amyloidosis. Recently, a new drug, tafamidis, has become available for TTR amyloid. It works by stabilizing transthyretin protein.

Cardiac biopsy is the reference standard for diagnosing CA; however, recent advances in echocardiography and MRI imaging have allowed for recognizing cardiac amyloid early. Diffuse endocardial gadolinium enhancements are characteristic findings in AL and TTR amyloid on cardiac MRI. A nuclear technetium pyrophosphate has become the gold standard for differentiating AL amyloid from TTR amyloid.[3] Decreased voltage on ECG relative to the amount of increased wall thickness on echocardiogram is typically seen.

Echocardiographic patterns of all forms of cardiac amyloid include increased LV and RV wall thickness, preserved LV systolic function, and atrial enlargement. Pericardial and pleural effusions may be present. Spectral Doppler evaluation typically demonstrates diastolic dysfunction with a restrictive pattern. Speckle tracking longitudinal strain shows regional sparing of the apical strain relative to the mid-wall and basal segments.[3] Relative regional strain ratio (RRSR), a measure of the degree of apical sparing of longitudinal strain, has been used to differentiate cardiac amyloidosis from other forms of LV hypertrophy. Other causes of LV hypertrophy such as uncontrolled hypertension, aortic stenosis, hypertrophic cardiomyopathies, and other forms of infiltrative cardiomyopathies should be ruled out. Cardiac amyloid may have features of hypertrophic cardiomyopathy including LV outflow gradient and systolic anterior motion of the mitral valve.[3]

References

3. Fazlinezhad A, Naqvi TZ. Cardiac amyloidosis: mimics, multimodality imaging diagnosis, and treatment. *JACC Cardiovasc Imaging.* 2020;13(6):1384-1391. doi:10.1016/j.jcmg.2019.12.014.

Case 4—A 56 Year Old Woman With Dyspnea and Chest Pain

History

A 56-year-old woman presented with shortness of breath going from one room to another (class III), symptoms varying from day to day. She reported exertional left shoulder pain. There was no history of palpitations, syncope, presyncope, or family history of sudden death. A coronary angiogram two years ago performed for shoulder pain did not reveal significant coronary artery disease (CAD).

Medications

Lisinopril 20 mg twice daily, labetalol 200 mg thrice daily, aspirin 81 mg, and amlodipine 5 mg once daily.

BP 170/100 mm Hg. Heart sounds were normal, S1 and S2 were present. Grade 2/6 to 3/6 ejection systolic murmur, best heard at the LV apex and the right parasternal area, which is accentuated with the Valsalva maneuver.

Electrocardiogram

Showed sinus rhythm with voltage criteria of left ventricular hypertrophy and repolarization changes (Fig. 9.24).

HHE was performed and showed proximal-to-mid IVS hypertrophy (Fig. 9.25 and Video 9.9), mild systolic anterior motion of the mitral valve (Fig. 9.25 and Video 9.9), prominent papillary muscles with mid-cavity obstruction (Fig. 9.26) and turbulent flow in mid-LV and LV outflow tract (Fig. 9.27 and Video 9.10).

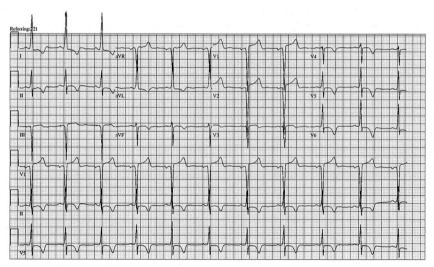

Fig. 9.24 Twelve-Lead ECG Showing Voltage Criteria for Left Ventricular Hypertrophy and Associated Repolarization Abnormalities of T Wave Inversion in Most Leads.

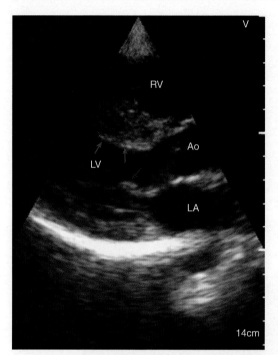

Fig. 9.25 HHE Parasternal Long-Axis View Showing Asymmetric Proximal Interventricular Septal Hypertrophy (yellow arrows) With Mild Systolic Anterior Motion of the Mitral Valve (red arrow). *Ao,* Aortic root; *LA,* left atrium; *LV,* left ventricle; *RV,* right ventricle.

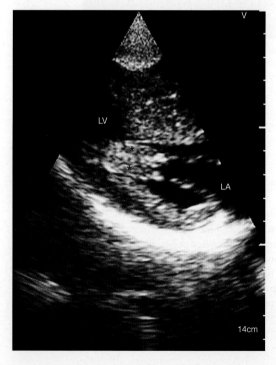

Fig. 9.26 HHE Off-Axis Parasternal Long-Axis View Showing Prominent and Somewhat Apically Displaced Posterior Papillary Muscle With Mid-Ventricular Crowding (double red asterisks). *LA,* Left atrium; *LV,* left ventricle.

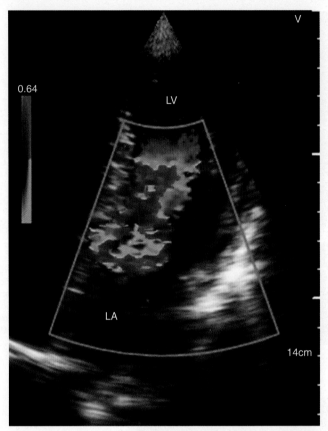

Fig. 9.27 HHE Apical 5-Chamber View With Color Doppler Showing Turbulent Color Doppler Flow in the Mid Ventricle and Left Ventricular Outflow Tract. *LA,* Left atrium; *LV,* left ventricle.

A standard echocardiogram after the consultation showed proximal IVS hypertrophy with systolic anterior motion of the mitral valve on M mode (Fig. 9.28) and apical three-chamber view (Fig. 9.29).

There was marked provocable LVOT gradient of 100 mm Hg (Fig. 9.30).

Clinical Management

As a result of vasodilator, effects lisinopril and amlodipine were discontinued and she was started on started verapamil 80 mg twice daily (subsequently converted to 240 mg once daily), metoprolol succinate 25 mg once daily, increased subsequently to 100 mg twice daily. At follow-up 3 months later, her dyspnea on exertion improved to NYHA class II along with resolution of exertional shoulder pain. Subsequently, provocable LVOT gradient of 100 mm Hg with Valsalva maneuver led to hospitalization for initiation of Disopyramide. She eventually underwent septal myomectomy because of recurrence of class II symptoms and LVOT gradient and achieved a marked improvement in symptoms and a marked decrease in LVOT gradient (Fig. 9.31).

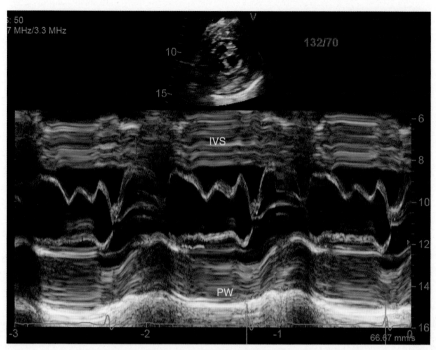

Fig. 9.28 M Mode Through Basal Short Axis Using Standard Echocardiogram Showing Systolic Anterior Motion of the Mitral Valve (yellow arrows). *IVS,* Interventricular septum; *PW,* posterior wall.

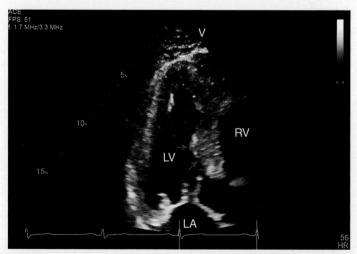

Fig. 9.29 Apical 3-Chamber View With a Standard Echocardiogram Showing Systolic Anterior Motion of the Mitral Valve (red arrow) and Hypertrophy of the Proximal Interventricular Septum (yellow arrows). *LA,* Left atrium; *LV,* left ventricle; *RV,* right ventricle.

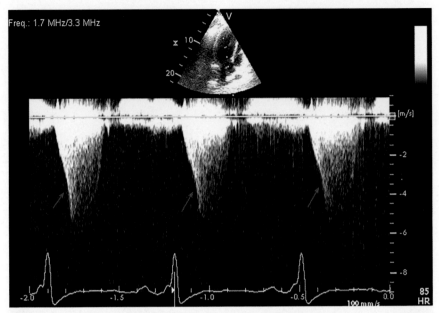

Fig. 9.30   Continuous-wave Doppler in the 3-chamber view across LV outflow tract using standard echocardiogram system showing a dagger-shaped late-peaking velocity of 5 m/sec (yellow arrows) corresponding to a gradient of 100 mm Hg.

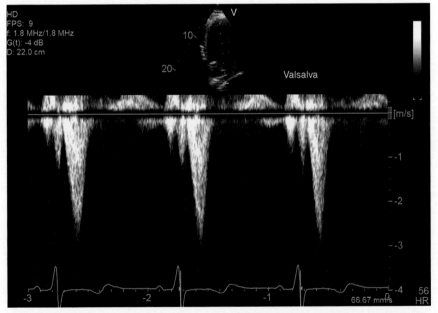

Fig. 9.31   Continuous-wave Doppler in the 3-chamber view across LV outflow tract using standard echocardiogram system after septal myomectomy showing significant decrease in provocable LVOT gradient with peak velocity of 2.7 m/s corresponding to a gradient of 29 mm Hg.

Teaching Point

Hypertrophic cardiomyopathy (HCM) is the most common heritable cardiomyopathy.[1] Left ventricular hypertrophy on echocardiogram in the absence of a secondary cause should make one consider HCM and infiltrative cardiomyopathy. ECG findings of LV hypertrophy concordant to echocardiographic LV hypertrophy help differentiate it from cardiac amyloid. The genetic mutations involve sarcomeric proteins; however, the specific underlying mutation may remain undetermined. Patient presentation ranges from asymptomatic to dyspnea, angina, heart failure, or sudden cardiac death.[1]

An increase in septal wall thickness, abnormal papillary muscle geometry, and abnormality of the mitral valve resulting in systolic anterior motion of the mitral valve collectively result in dynamic left ventricular outflow obstruction in most patients. The goal of therapeutic interventions is largely to reduce dynamic obstruction. Lifestyle modifications such as preventing dehydration, weight loss, control of hypertension, rate slowing medications, and medications with negative inotropic effects are the main pharmacotherapies. Disopyramide is added if intraventricular obstruction and symptoms persist. Alcohol septal ablation and septal reduction surgery are other options. Both are effective in reducing/eliminating gradients; however, surgery is associated with a better long-term outcome when performed at a center of excellence (Fig. 9.32).[1] Recently tested new pharmacologic treatment with a cardiac myosin inhibitor, mavacamten, has shown a marked reduction in obstructive gradient and quality of life in patients with obstructive HCM.[2]

A small subset of patients with HCM will experience sudden cardiac death. Septal wall thickness >3 cm, a history of syncope, family history of sudden cardiac death, nonsustained VT on Holter monitor, and the presence of fibrosis on MRI of >20% are associated with increased risk of sudden cardiac death; however, risk stratification remains a clinical challenge.

Transthoracic echocardiography remains the mainstay of cardiac imaging in HCM. Severity and distribution of LVH, presence of systolic anterior motion (SAM) of the mitral valve, eccentric posteriorly directed MR jet secondary to SAM, and LVOT late-peaking dagger-shaped gradient that increases with the Valsalva maneuver are the main abnormalities to evaluate. LVH is the hallmark of HCM diagnosis. LVH severity plays an important role in prognostication and SCD risk assessment decision making. Strain assessment provides additional insights into myocardial disarray.

Final Diagnosis

Hypertrophic obstructive cardiomyopathy was the definitive diagnosis.

The Role of HHE in Clinical Management

HHE showed features of hypertrophic obstructive cardiomyopathy, which were subsequently confirmed with a standard echocardiogram.

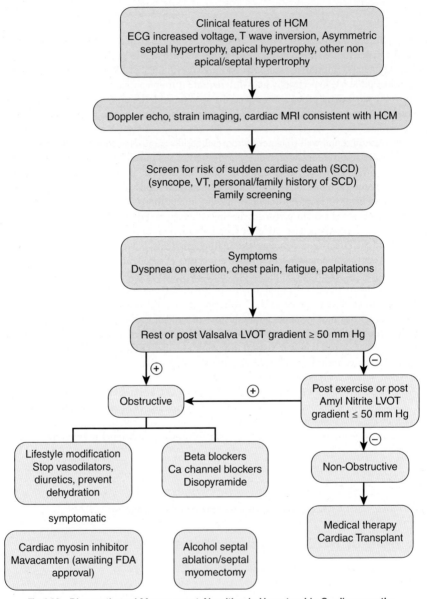

Fig. 9.32   Diagnostic and Management Algorithm in Hypertrophic Cardiomyopathy.

References

1. Geske JB, Ommen SR, Gersh BJ, et al. Hypertrophic cardiomyopathy clinical update. *JACC Heart Fail.* 2018;6(5):364-375.
2. Ho CY, Olivotto I, Jacoby D, et al. Evaluation of mavacamten in adults with symptomatic obstructive hypertrophic cardiomyopathy. *Circ Heart Fail.* 2020;13(6):e006853. doi:10.1161/CIRCHEARTFAILURE. 120.006853.

CHAPTER 10

Case 1—62-Year-Old Man for General Medical Evaluation

History

A 62-year-old man presented for routine general medical evaluation. There was a history of mild exertional dyspnea and palpitations. His New York Heart Association class was class I. There was no abnormal heart rate or rhythm on Apple Watch 5 monitoring.

Physical Examination

Physical examination undertaken by an outside cardiologist 4 months ago had revealed a "murmur." Stress echocardiogram was performed. Exercise capacity was 10 metabolic equivalents (METS). Stress echocardiogram was negative for ischemia but did show severe mitral valve regurgitation (MR) and left atrial enlargement. Resting blood pressure was 150/80 mm Hg.

Laboratory Values

- Normal complete blood count (CBC), basic metabolic panel, and liver function tests (LFTs) were recorded.
- N-terminal proB-type natriuretic peptide, NT-proBNP: 110 pg/mL (normal 10-82 pg/mL).
- ECG was normal.

Chest Radiography

Chest x-ray (CXR) showed mild cardiomegaly and pulmonary venous congestion (Fig. 10.1).

Handheld Echocardiography Findings

- HHE during consultation demonstrated mildly increased end-diastolic and normal (2.9 cm) left ventricular end-systolic diameter (LVESD) and ejection fraction (LVEF) >60% (Fig. 10.2, Video 10.1); left atrial enlargement; flail P2 scallop of posterior mitral leaflet with torn chords in the parasternal long axis (Figs. 10.2 and 10.3, Video 10.1), short axis, (Fig. 10.4, Video 10.2), and apical four-chamber view (Fig. 10.5, Video 10.3) with severe MR (Fig. 9.6, Video 10.4). Standard TTE showed left ventricular end-diastolic diameter (LVEDD) of 62 mm, LVEF of 66%, and severe MR with flail P2 scallop.

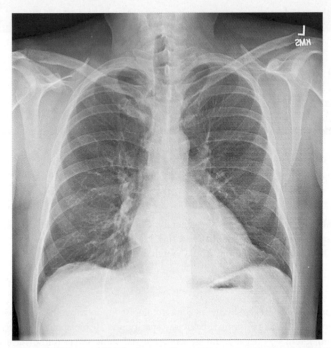

Fig. 10.1   CXR Showing Mild Cardiomegaly and Pulmonary Venous Congestion.

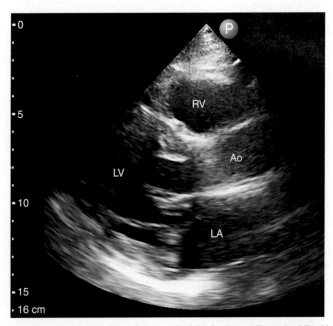

Fig. 10.2   HHE Parasternal Long-Axis View Showing Flail P2 Scallop of Posterior Mitral Leaflet (yellow arrow). There is a mild increase in left ventricular *(LV)* end-diastolic and left atrial diameters. *Ao,* Aortic root; *LA,* left atrium; *RV,* right ventricle.

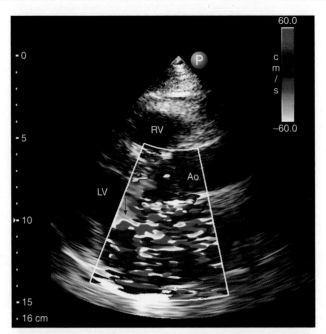

Fig. 10.3 HHE Parasternal Long-Axis Color Doppler View Showing Mitral Regurgitation Jet Filling the Left Atrium With Proximal Flow Acceleration at a Normal Aliasing Velocity of 60 cm/s Suggesting the Presence of Severe MR (red arrow). *Ao,* Aortic root; *LV,* left ventricle; *RV,* right ventricle.

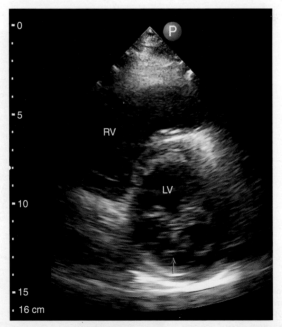

Fig. 10.4 HHE Short-Axis View at the Mitral Valve Level Showing a Myxomatous Mitral Valve With Posterior Leaflet Prolapse (yellow arrow). *LV,* Left ventricle; *RV,* right ventricle.

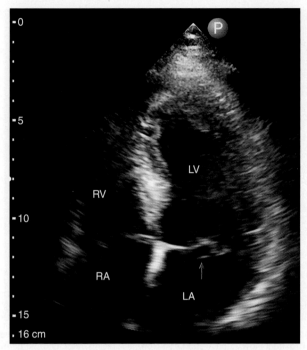

Fig. 10.5 HHE Apical 4-Chamber View Showing a Torn Chord Protruding into the Left Atrium *(LA)* **(yellow arrow).** *LV,* Left ventricle; *RA,* Right atrium; *RV,* right ventricle.

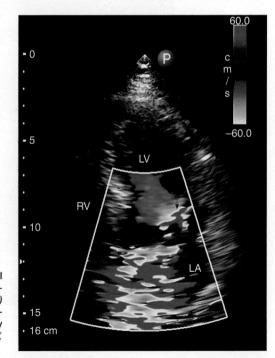

Fig. 10.6 HHE Color Doppler Apical 4-Chamber View Showing Severe Mitral Regurgitation Jet Filling Up the Left Atrium *(LA)* and With a Large Proximal Flow Acceleration (red arrow) at Normal Aliasing Velocity of 60 cm/s. LVEF was approximately 65%. *LV,* Left ventricle; *RV,* right ventricle.

Subsequent Course

- The treatment approaches of watchful waiting and early surgical mitral valve repair were considered. The patient was started on losartan 50 mg and hydrochlorothiazide 12.5 mg for hypertension.
- The risk for MR recurrence after mitral valve repair was discussed, along with data on the increased incidence of sudden death in patients with flail mitral leaflet who are managed with watchful waiting.
- The physician decided to do a transesophageal echocardiogram (TEE) to evaluate mitral valve anatomy and potential surgical success rate for repair.

Transesophageal Echocardiogram

TEE confirmed P2 flail (Fig. 10.7) and a single jet of severe, eccentric, anterior-directed mitral regurgitation (Fig. 10.8). Three-dimensional (3D) echocardiogram showed flail of the entire P2 scallop with multiple torn chords (Fig. 10.9).

Clinical Course

- The patient requested robot-assisted mitral valve repair.
- The surgeon requested CT angiograms of the chest, abdomen, and pelvis for determining the feasibility of robot-assisted mitral valve repair surgery.
- CT imaging showed no significant coronary disease and confirmed echocardiographic findings of flail of the posterior leaflet.

Subsequent Course

- Patient underwent robotic mitral valve repair surgery with triangular resection of the medial portion of a large P2 scallop with multiple torn chords.
- Mitral valve repair was successfully performed with a 63-mm Medtronic band. Suture repair of a patent foramen ovale (PFO) was also performed.

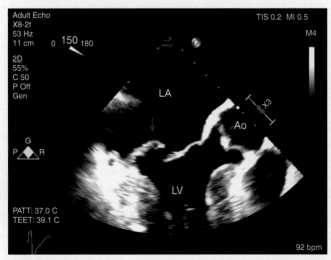

Fig. 10.7 2D TEE 3-Chamber View Showing Flail of the Posterior Mitral Leaflet (yellow arrow). *Ao*, Aortic root; *LA*, left atrium; *LV*, left ventricle.

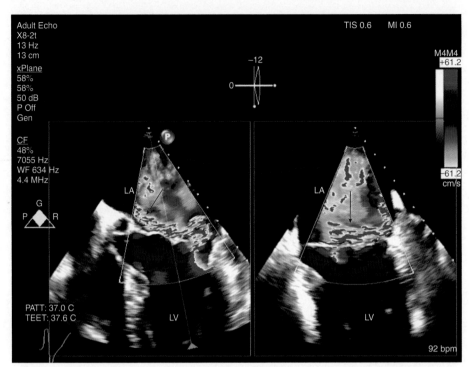

Fig. 10.8 TEE biplane Color Doppler View Showing Eccentric Severe Anteriorly Directed MR (red arrows) Jet in the 4-Chamber (left) and 2-Chamber Views (right). *LA,* Left atrium; *LV,* left ventricle.

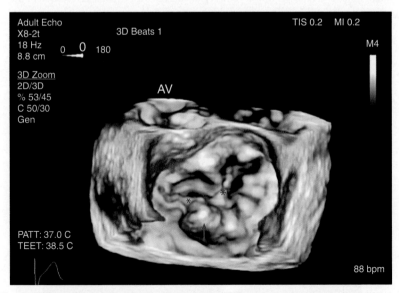

Fig. 10.9 3D TEE Images Acquired in the "Zoom Mode." Mitral valve is shown from the atrial perspective in the "surgeon's view." Aortic valve *(AV)* is on top at the 11 o'clock position. Flail of large P2 scallop (yellow arrow) along with thorn chords *(red asterisks)* are shown.

Final Diagnosis

Flail P2 scallop of the posterior mitral valve leaflet with severe mitral regurgitation.

Utility of HHE in Clinical Management

HHE helped diagnose flail of the posterior leaflet with severe MR with normal LV size and ejection fraction during first outpatient visit.

Teaching Point

- Determinants of Timing of Corrective Surgery in Primary Mitral Regurgitation.[1]
  - The optimal timing of corrective surgery is determined by a number of factors, including:
    1. MR severity
    2. Presence or absence of symptoms
    3. Functional state of the left ventricle
    4. Feasibility of valve repair
    5. Presence of atrial fibrillation
    6. Presence of pulmonary hypertension at rest or with exercise
    7. Preference and expectations of the patient
- Mitral Valve Repair in Asymptomatic Severe MR with Degenerative Mitral Valve Disease
  - Mitral valve repair is reasonable in asymptomatic patients with chronic severe primary MR (stage C1) and preserved LV function (LVEF >60% and LVESD <40 mm) in whom the likelihood of a successful and durable repair without residual MR is greater than 95% with an expected mortality rate of less than 1% when performed at a Heart Valve Center of Excellence.

Reference

1. Nishimura RA, Otto CA, Bonow RO, et al. AHA/ACC focused update of the 2014 AHA/ACC guideline for the management of patients with valvular heart disease: a report of the American College of Cardiology/American Heart Association Task Force on Clinical Practice Guidelines. *Circulation*. 2017;135:e1159–e1195.

Case 2—An 81-Year-Old Man Undergoing Workup for Transcutaneous Aortic Valve Replacement (TAVR) for Severe Aortic Stenosis Presents With Severe Dyspnea

History

An 81-year-old man with known severe calcific aortic stenosis (AS) undergoing workup for transcatheter aortic valve replacement (TAVR) presented to the emergency room with a 4-day history of severe shortness of breath and multiple episodes of paroxysmal nocturnal dyspnea. He denied any chest pain.

Past medical history was significant for nonalcoholic hepatic cirrhosis complicated by hepatocellular carcinoma treated with radiation therapy and remission free for >5 years.

Physical Examination

Physical examination revealed: HR, 86 bpm; blood pressure, 124/74 mm Hg; O_2 saturation over 95% on 2 L nasal cannula; mild elevation of jugular venous pressure (JVP); a 4/6 crescendo-decrescendo systolic murmur at the R second intercostal space, with radiation to both carotid arteries; a slow rising carotid upstroke as well as bibasilar crackles; extending to R-mid zone; and reduced breath sounds at the base of the left lung.

A diagnosis of congestive heart failure (CHF) was made secondary to underlying severe aortic stenosis, or new onset paroxysmal tachyarrhythmia, or an acute coronary syndrome.

Handheld Echocardiography

A HHE was performed in the emergency room after initial evaluation. Parasternal long-axis view showed akinesis of mid-to-distal anterior interventricular septum with reduced LVEF estimated at 35% (Fig. 10.10, Video 10.5). There was hypokinesis of distal inferior IVS, distal inferior, and anterior walls, and dyskinesis of LV apex. RV function and RA pressure were normal.

These wall motion abnormalities were new compared with a prior standard echocardiogram performed 2 weeks before presentation, which had shown a normal LVEF of 65% and no regional wall motion abnormalities (Fig. 10.11) with severe AS and a mean gradient of 55 mm Hg. An ECG (Fig. 10.12) showed new changes from prior ECGs (Fig. 10.13) with ST elevation in leads V1-V4.

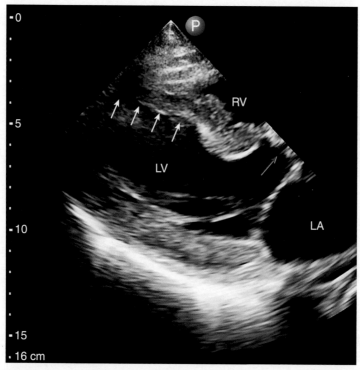

Fig. 10.10 HHE Parasternal Long-Axis End-Systolic View Showing Dilation of Left Ventricle *(LV)* and Akinesis of Mid-To-Distal Interventricular Septum (white arrows) and Calcified Aortic Valve (yellow arrow). *LA,* Left atrium; *RV,* right ventricle.

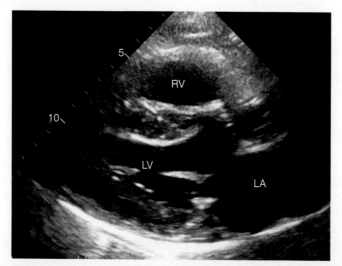

Fig. 10.11 Standard Echocardiogram of Parasternal Long-Axis End-Systolic View Before Current Presentation Showing Normal Left Ventricle; *(LV)* End-Systolic Size With Normal Interventricular Septal Thickening. *LA,* Left atrium; *RV,* right ventricle.

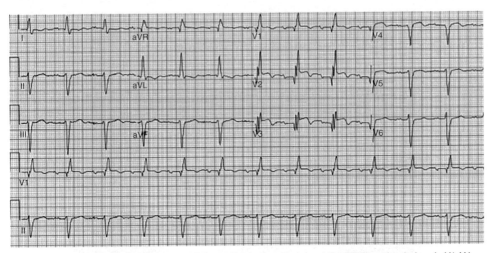

Fig. 10.12 Twelve-Lead ECG Obtained After HHE Imaging Showing Mild ST Elevation in Leads V1-V4 Q waves in leads V2-V4, and decreased R Waves in the Remaining Precordial Leads.

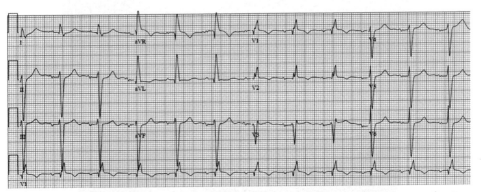

Fig. 10.13 Twelve-Lead ECG before Current Presentation Showing Sinus Rhythm, Right Bundle Branch Block, and Associated T Wave Inversions in Leads V1 and V2.

An angiogram had been performed 3 weeks ago performed for TAVR workup had shown a 90% proximal left anterior descending artery (LAD) lesion at the origin of the first diagonal coronary artery (Fig. 10.14) and a 90% mid-right coronary artery (RCA) stenosis. Subsequently, laboratory data became available.

Laboratory Data Obtained in the Emergency Room

Troponin 115 (n ≤ 15 ng/L)
Normal creatinine clearance
N-terminal proB-type natriuretic peptide, NT-proBNP 8268 pg/mL (n < 325 pg/mL)

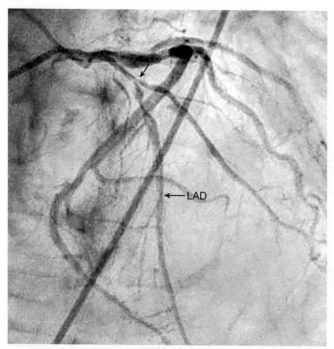

Fig. 10.14 Selective Left Coronary Angiography Before Current Presentation Showing Severe LAD Stenosis at the Origin of the First Diagonal Branch (red arrow).

Clinical Course

Based on the findings on HHE, a significant change from a recent echocardiogram, new ECG changes, and elevated troponin, the patient was sent to the cardiac catheterization laboratory for percutaneous coronary intervention (PCI). A bare-metal stent was placed in the proximal LAD lesion along with balloon angioplasty of ostial first diagonal lesion. There was a 90% mid-RCA lesion, which was not intervened on. Bare metal stent was placed due to uncertainty regarding need for subsequent CABG. Twenty-four hours later maximum troponin was 331 ng/L.

Standard TTE was performed after coronary intervention 24 hours after presentation showed persistent akinesis of mid-to-distal interventricular septum (IVS). Apical four-chamber microbubble-enhanced apical images showed dyskinetic LV apex and distal LV segments without an LV thrombus (Fig. 10.15, Video 10.6). LVEF was 40%.

During bedside round 36 hours later, an HHE was done to evaluate for presence of pleural effusions as a result of physical examination findings and the patient's complaint of dyspnea. Bilateral pleural effusions were found, a smaller R and a larger L pleural effusion (Fig. 10.16 and Video 10.7). The patient underwent left pleurocentesis with removal of 800 cc of transudative fluid with and had a marked symptomatic improvement in dyspnea after the procedure. Next day 800 mL of transudative R pleural fluid was tapped and the patient had a further symptomatic improvement in dyspnea.

A cardiac magnetic resonance imaging (MRI) performed 24 hours later showed LAD distribution ischemia/infarction with remodeling and focal hypokinesis in the anterior and anteroseptal mid-to-apical ventricle, and LVEF was 42%. Delayed enhancement was noted in the mid-to-distal anteroseptal segment only.

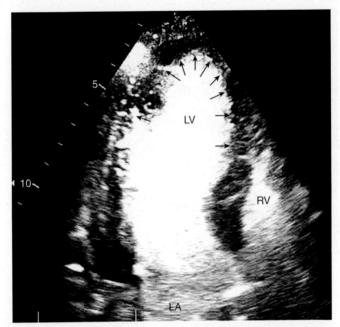

Fig. 10.15 Standard TTE Microbubble-Enhanced End-Systolic Apical 4-Chamber View Showing True LV Apex With Dyskinesis Extending to Neighboring Distal LV Segments and Reduced Thickening of Mid-LV Segments (black arrows). *LA,* Left atrium; *LV,* left ventricle; *RV,* right ventricle.

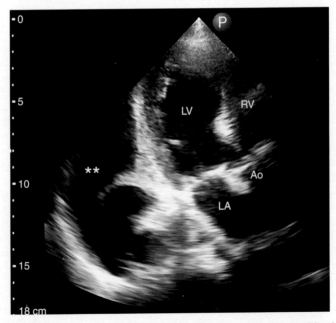

Fig. 10.16 HHE Apical 3-Chamber View Showing a Large Left Pleural Effusion (double white asterisks). *Ao,* Aortic root; *LA,* left atrium; *LV,* left ventricle; *RV,* right ventricle.

Subsequent Clinical Course

Due to a lack of viability in the infarcted LAD segments, a decistion was made to perform TAVR instead of surgical AVR. Patient underwent transfemoral TAVR with a 29-mm Sapien 3 valve (Edwards Lifesciences, Irvine, California) 4 weeks later along with an RCA stent. LVEF improved to 45% after TAVR on a standard echocardiogram. Patient needed a periprocedural pacemaker.

Final Diagnosis

Acute LAD territory myocardial infarction in a patient with severe aortic stenosis, with moderate LV systolic dysfunction and CHF treated with emergent PCI and subsequent TAVR.

Utility of Handheld Echocardiography in Patient Management

Handheld echocardiography confirmed new regional wall motion abnormalities in the LAD territory and significant reduction in LV function from a recent echocardiogram. A diagnosis of acute myocardial infarction (AMI) was made, and the patient was sent to the cardiac catheterization laboratory. HHE subsequently confirmed pleural effusions as the etiology of subsequent dyspnea, which improved after bilateral pleurocentesis.

Teaching Point

At the present time, the choice of proceeding with surgical AVR versus TAVR is based on multiple factors, including the surgical risk, patient frailty, comorbid conditions, and patient preferences and values. Concomitant severe coronary artery disease may also affect the optimal intervention, because severe multivessel coronary disease may best be served by surgical AVR and coronary artery bypass graft surgery (CABG).

The prevalence of coronary artery disease (CAD) in TAVR patients ranges from 40% to 75%.[1] The influence of CAD in TAVR recipients remains controversial, and no definite data exist on the most appropriate revascularization strategy or the appropriate timing of PCI.[2] Because TAVR can cause hemodynamic instability and increased myocardial supply-demand mismatch during rapid pacing and balloon inflation, left ventricular outflow tract obstruction from the delivery catheter and hypotension from anesthesia present a high ischemic burden, especially with diminished left ventricular function. Proximal LAD or left main lesions are often treated with selective revascularization either before or, more commonly, during TAVR procedures. At present, a lesion in the proximal LAD, significant CAD (measured by fractional flow reserve if needed) and large ischemia burden are treated with coronary revascularization before or during TAVR. Although PCI may relieve symptomatic CAD, oftentimes symptomatic AS may be difficult to differentiate from symptomatic CAD. However, there is no randomized trial to date comparing this strategy versus no revascularization.

Apical foreshortening of images may miss LV apical abnormalities such as dyskinesis or apical thrombus, and microbubble-enhanced echocardiogram provides better evaluation of LV apical segments.

References

1. Goel SS, Ige M, Tuzcu EM, et al. Severe aortic stenosis and coronary artery disease-implications for management in the transcatheter aortic valve replacement era: a comprehensive review. *J Am Coll Cardiol.* 2013;62:1-10.
2. Faroux L, Guimaraes L, Wintzer-Wehekind J, et al. Coronary artery disease and transcatheter aortic valve replacement. JACC state-of-the-art review. *J Am Coll Cardiol.* 2019;74(3):362-372.

Case 3—Incidental Finding on CT Chest Screening for Lung Cancer in a 56-Year-Old Woman

History

- A 56-year-old Caucasian woman underwent chest CT for lung cancer screening for smoking. CT findings suggestive of pulmonary hypertension led to cardiology outpatient referral. NYHA class was II
- Past medical history was significant for bronchitis and stage 3 chronic renal disease with estimated glomerular filtration rate of 30 to 59 mL/m²/min.
- Patient has no history of rheumatic fever and was raised in the US.

Physical Examination

- Sinus rhythm was present with a heart rate of 95 bpm.
- There was a 4/6 holosystolic murmur of mitral regurgitation and a short diastolic murmur without an opening snap at the cardiac apex. There was a loud P2 over the pulmonic area.
- No crackles or rales were heard.

Electrocardiography

ECG showed sinus rhythm and mild RV strain pattern (Fig. 10.17).

Chest Radiography

CXR showed mild cardiomegaly with straightening of left border, prominent branch pulmonary arteries, and mild pulmonary congestion (Fig. 10.18).

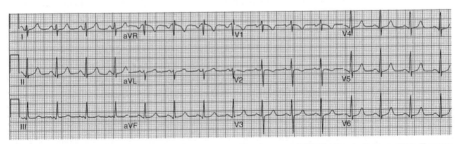

Fig. 10.17 Twelve-Lead ECG Showing Normal Sinus Rhythm and Mild RV Strain Pattern With T wave Inversions in V1 and V2 and Prominent R in V2.

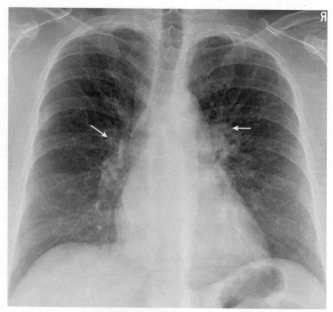

Fig. 10.18 Chest Radiograph Showing Mild Cardiomegaly With Straightening of Left Heart Border, Prominent Pulmonary Arteries (white arrows), and Pulmonary Venous Congestion.

Handheld Echocardiography

An HHE was performed during office consultation. Parasternal long-axis view showed a hyperkinetic LV with dilated RV outflow tract, dilated left atrium, and diffusely thickened and noncalcified mitral valve anterior and posterior leaflets with restricted leaflet opening and malcoaptation (Fig. 10.19, Video 10.8). Color Doppler showed severe mitral regurgitation jet originating at the center and directed posteriorly (Figs. 10.20A-B, Video 10.9). Short-axis view showed hyperkinetic LV with mild flattening of IVS, dilated RV, thickening of mitral valve leaflets with marked posterior leaflet restriction, minimal anterolateral commissural fusion, and no posteromedial commissural fusion. Apical 4-chamber view showed a hyperkinetic LV, dilated left atrium, diffusely thickened mitral valve leaflets with malcoaptation, and fixed posterior mitral valve leaflet (Figs. 10.21A-B, Video 10.10). Color Doppler in the 4-chamber view showed severe mitral regurgitation (Fig. 10.22). In addition, there was diastolic turbulence at a normal aliasing velocity of 0.64 m/sec across the mitral valve on color Doppler, suggestive of significant mitral stenosis (Fig. 10.20, Video 10.8). Subcostal view showed a small and collapsing inferior vena cava.

The patient denied history of diet drug use or intake of ergot or its derivatives, and there was no history of connective tissue disorder. A previous antinuclear antibody test was negative. Presence of mixed mitral valve disease and disease severity were discussed with the patient along with further diagnostic workup and the need for mitral valve surgery. The patient did not want to take lifelong anticoagulation medications.

Standard TTE confirmed HHE findings. Mean mitral valve gradient was 14 mm Hg (at HR of 97 bpm), mitral valve area (MVA) was 0.87 cm^2 by continuity equation, peak pulmonary artery pressure was 76 mm Hg and severe MR was confirmed. A TEE was performed and showed

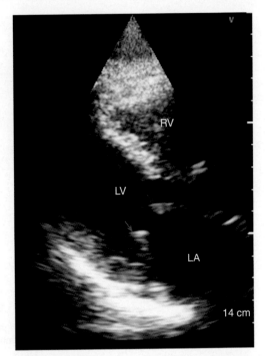

Fig. 10.19 HHE Parasternal Long-Axis View Showing Diffusely Thickened and Noncalcified Mitral Valve Anterior (red arrow) and Posterior Leaflets (yellow arrow) With Restricted Leaflet Opening and Dilated Left Atrium. *LA,* Left atrium; *LV,* left ventricle; *RV,* right ventricle.

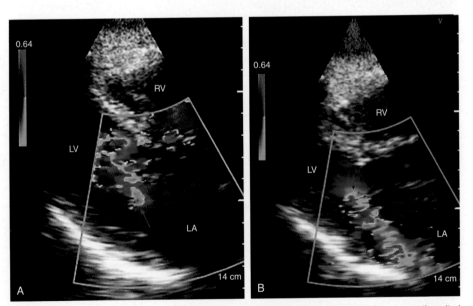

Fig. 10.20   (A) HHE parasternal long axis diastolic color Doppler view showing turbulent flow across the mitral valve (yellow arrow). (B) HHE parasternal long axis color systolic Doppler view showing severe mitral regurgitation (red arrow). *LA,* Left atrium; *LV,* left ventricle; *RV,* right ventricle.

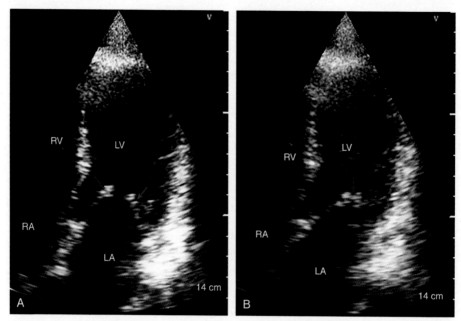

Fig. 10.21   (A) HHE apical 4-chamber view in diastole showing thickened anterior (red arrow) and posterior (yellow arrow) mitral valve leaflets with restricted opening during diastole and markedly enlarged left atrium *(LA)*. (B) HHE apical 4-chamber view in end systole showing mitral leaflet thickening and malcoaptation (green arrow). *LV*, Left ventricle; *RA*, right atrium; *RV*, right ventricle.

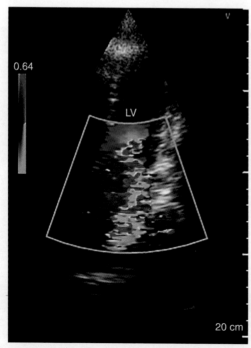

Fig. 10.22   **HHE Apical 4-Chamber View in End Systole Showing Severe Mitral Regurgitation.** *LV*, Left ventricle.

diffusely thickened and restricted mitral valve leaflets (Figs. 10.23 and 10.24), severe MR (Fig. 10.24), moderate right ventricular enlargement with mild hypokinesis and short, thickened, and fused mitral chordae. Three-dimensional (3D) imaging showed thickened mitral valve leaflets with marked posterior leaflet restriction, mild commissural fusion, and leaflet malcoaptation (Figs. 10.25A-B). There was no left atrial appendage thrombus.

Cardiac Catheterization Report

The patient was subsequently referred for right and left heart catheterization, which showed:
- Pulmonary capillary wedge pressure 32, V wave up to 45 mm Hg
- PA pressure 92/45 mm Hg
- RV pressure 90/14 mm Hg
- RA mean pressure 10 mm Hg.

Coronary angiogram showed a 30% obstructive lesion in the RCA, which disappeared after nitroglycerin administration.

A diagnosis of Type II pulmonary hypertension (secondary to left heart disease) was made, and the patient was referred to CT surgery for mitral valve replacement.

Subsequent Clinical Course

- Patient underwent mitral valve replacement 42 days later with a 29-mm Medtronic mosaic porcine mitral valve prosthesis.
- Surgical findings showed marked mitral leaflet and chordal thickening and moderate chordal fusion.
- Pathology showed advanced postinflammatory (possibly rheumatic) fibrotic mitral valve disease.

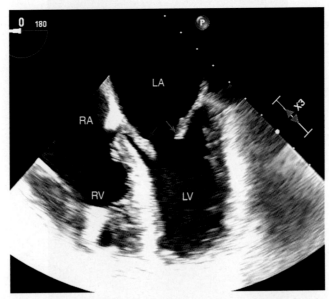

Fig. 10.23   Transesophageal Echocardiographic 4-Chamber View in Diastole Showing Anterior (red arrow) and Posterior (yellow arrow) Mitral Leaflet Thickening, Dilated Right Ventricle and Biatrial Enlargement. *LA,* Left atrium; *LV,* left ventricle; *RA,* right atrium; *RV,* right ventricle.

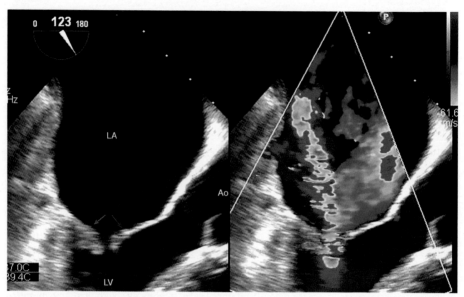

Fig. 10.24 Transesophageal Echocardiographic 3-Chamber View in End Systole Showing Anterior (red arrow) and Posterior (yellow arrow) Mitral Leaflet Thickening, Restriction, Leaflet Malcoaptation (left panel), and Severe Mitral Regurgitation (right panel). The left atrium is severely enlarged. *LA,* Left atrium; *LV,* left ventricle.

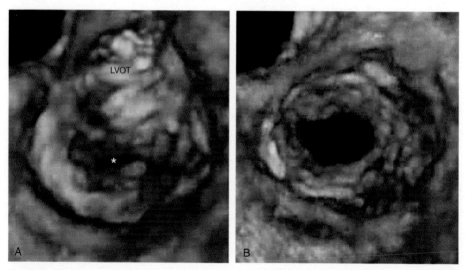

Fig. 10.25 (A) 3D transesophageal view from the ventricular perspective showing anterior (red arrow) and posterior (yellow arrow) mitral leaflet thickening and malcoaptation in end systole (white asterisk). (B) 3D transesophageal view from the ventricular perspective showing mitral leaflet thickening and restricted leaflet opening in end diastole. *LVOT,* Left ventricular outflow tract.

Utility of Handheld Echocardiography in Patient Management

HHE demonstrated mitral leaflet thickening and restriction of leaflets with severe mitral regurgitation, right ventricular enlargement, and normal left ventricular function at the time of initial cardiac consultation.

Final Diagnosis

Postinflammatory mixed mitral valve disease was diagnosed.

Teaching Point

Majority of inflammatory mitral valve diseases are rheumatic in etiology. Other rare causes include intake of serotonergic drugs such as diet drugs, ergot and its derivatives for migraine, and carcinoid disease. The latter affects the right-sided valves unless there is a patent foramen ovale or there is primary lung carcinoid tumor. Rheumatic mitral valve diseases are comprised of leaflet fibrosis with restriction of leaflets, which is most marked in the posterior leaflet; commissural fusion and thickening; and fusion and shortening of subvalvular chordae tendineae. The most common presentation of rheumatic mitral valve disease is predominant mitral valve stenosis, although predominant mitral regurgitation or mixed mitral valve stenosis and regurgitation, as in our patient, are not uncommon presentations. Thickening, mobility, and calcification of mitral leaflets; shortening and thickening of chords; and presence of severity of mitral regurgitation determine treatment options such as percutaneous or surgical repair or replacement.

CHAPTER 11

Case 1—An 85-Year-Old Man With Remote Aortic Valve Replacement Presents With Dyspnea

History

An 85-year-old man presented with dyspnea on exertion, ankle swelling, and NYHA class II heart failure. He reported no orthopnea or paroxysmal nocturnal dyspnea. Patient had a bioprosthetic aortic valve (AV) implanted 15 years ago and was referred for "diastolic heart failure."

Physical Examination

There was a 3/6 crescendo-decrescendo systolic murmur at the right second intercostal space and a 3/6 holosystolic murmur at the cardiac apex. No diastolic murmur was audible. There was 1+ bilateral lower extremity pitting edema to just above ankles.

Electrocardiography

ECG showed sinus rhythm with voltage criteria of LV hypertrophy in the precordial leads.

Chest Radiography

Chest x-ray (CXR) showed a normal cardiac silhouette, blunting of the right costophrenic angle, sternotomy wires, and a bioprosthetic aortic valve.

Handheld Echocardiography Findings During Consultation

- Normal-to-hyperkinetic left ventricle with an ejection fraction estimated at 65% (Fig. 11.1, Video 11.1) and left ventricular hypertrophy.
- Mild-to-moderate right ventricular enlargement with interventricular septal (IVS) flattening (Fig. 11.1, Video 11.1).
- Marked mitral annular calcification extending to mitral leaflets (Fig. 11.1, Video 11.1) with markedly turbulent color Doppler flow across the mitral valve, moderate central mitral regurgitation, and left atrial enlargement (Fig. 11.2, Video 11.2).
- Moderate tricuspid regurgitation and marked right atrial enlargement.
- Bioprosthetic aortic valve with marked leaflet thickening and limited excursion, focal nodular calcification with possible mobile density on aortic cusp (Fig. 11.3, Video 11.3).
- There was an increase in right atrial (RA) pressure based on inferior vena cava (IVC) size estimated at 8 mm Hg.

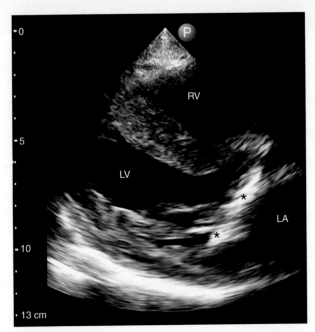

Fig. 11.1   HHE parasternal long-axis view showing thickening and calcification of bioprosthetic aortic valve (yellow arrow) and heavy mitral annular calcification (black asterisks). Dilated right venricle (RV) with interventricular septal flattening from RV pressure/volume overload is also shown. *LA,* Left atrium; *LV,* left ventricle.

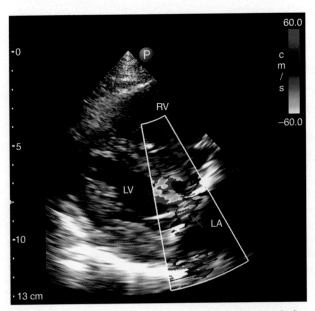

Fig. 11.2   HHE color Doppler parasternal long-axis view showing turbulent diastolic flow across the mitral valve suggestive of calcific mitral stenosis. *LA,* Left atrium; *LV,* left ventricle; *RV,* right ventricle.

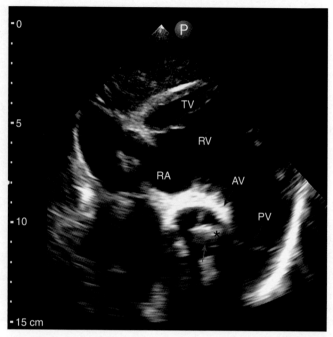

Fig. 11.3 HHE subcostal image in diastole showing tricuspid, bioprosthetic, and pulmonic valves (red arrows). There is calcification (black asterisk) and a nodular density on the aortic valve (AV) (yellow arrow). Dilated right ventricle (RV) inflow and outflow and dilated right atrium are also shown. *PV,* Pulmonic valve; *RA,* right atrium; *TV,* tricuspid valve.

Standard Echocardiogram

Standard echocardiogram confirmed bioprosthetic aortic valve (AV) stenosis (Fig. 11.4) with a mean AV gradient of 32 mm Hg (Fig. 11.5). Peak pulmonary artery (PA) pressure was 75 mm Hg, consistent with severe pulmonary hypertension. An outside echocardiogram 1 year ago had shown a mean AV gradient of 20 mm Hg.

Transesophageal Echocardiography

- A transesophageal echocardiogram (TEE) confirmed bioprosthetic aortic valve stenosis with cusp motion of the noncoronary cusp and fixed right coronary cusp of the aortic valve (Fig. 11.6). There was mild intravalvular regurgitation. Thrombus on AV could not be ruled out. Three-dimensional (3D) imaging of the mitral valve showed heavy mitral leaflet calcification (Fig. 11.7). Mean mitral valve gradient was 8 mm Hg (Fig. 11.8).

Subsequent Clinical Course

- A nodular thickening was found adjacent to valve leaflet calcification of the bioprosthetic AV, and an increase in AV gradient compared with a year ago was concerning for a possible valve thrombus. However, as a result of an increased serum creatinine of 2.5 mg/dL a contrast enhanced CT was not performed to rule out valve thrombosis.

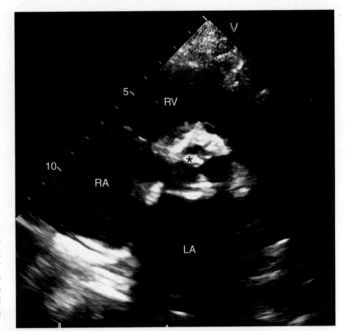

Fig. 11.4 Standard echo subcostal image in diastole showed calcification (black asterisk) as well as a nodular density on the Aortic valve (AV) Dilated right ventricle (RV) inflow and outflow and dilated right (RA) and left (LA) atria are also shown.

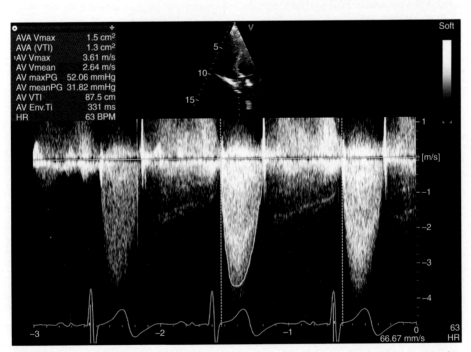

AVA Vmax	1.5 cm²
AVA (VTI)	1.3 cm²
AV Vmax	3.61 m/s
AV Vmean	2.64 m/s
AV maxPG	52.06 mmHg
AV meanPG	31.82 mmHg
AV VTI	87.5 cm
AV Env.Ti	331 ms
HR	63 BPM

Fig. 11.5 Standard TTE CW Doppler across the bioprosthetic aortic valve in the apical 3-chamber view showing peak and mean gradients of 52 mm Hg and 32 mm Hg respectively.

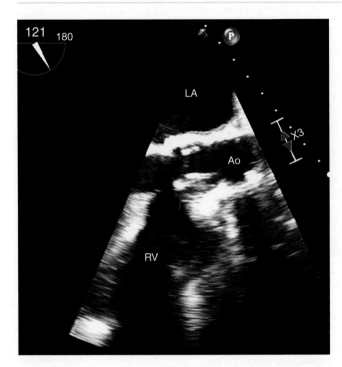

Fig. 11.6 2D TEE long-axis view in mid systole showing bioprosthetic aortic valve and aortic root (Ao). Normal non-coronary cusp motion seen in fully open position (red arrow). There is restricted motion, thickening and calcification at the site of the right coronary cusp of the bioprosthetic aortic valve (yellow arrow). *LA,* Left atrium; *RV,* right ventricle.

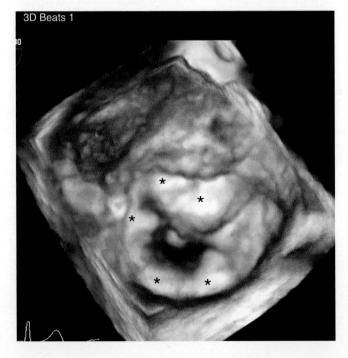

Fig. 11.7 3D TEE image of the mitral valve from the atrial perspective showing heavy mitral annular calcification (black asterisks) encroaching onto the anterior and posterior leaflets and causing calcific mitral stenosis. Aortic valve is located at the 12 o'clock position.

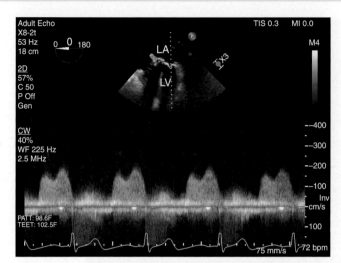

Fig. 11.8   2D TEE CW Doppler across the mitral valve in the 4-chamber views showing mitral inflow mean gradient of 8 mm Hg at a HR of 72 bpm suggestive of significant calcific mitral stenosis. *LA*, Left atrium; *LV*, left ventricle.

- The patient was started on a trial of coumadin with an international normalized ratio (INR) goal of 2 to 3 with a plan for follow-up assessment of AV gradient and nodular thickening.
- Metoprolol dose was increased from 50 to 62.5 mg a day to allow for a slower heart rate and reduced mitral gradient. Renal insufficiency and mixed mitral stenosis and regurgitation were considered to be the etiology of pulmonary hypertension. Furosemide was increased.
- Patient presented with a gastrointestinal bleed 3.5 weeks later and coumadin was stopped. No change in AV gradient occurred when the patient was on coumadin.
- Subsequent capsule endoscopy and CT enterography identified a small bowel mass that was found to be diffusely metastatic on subsequent positron emission tomography CT scan, and the patient died 5 months later.

Utility of Handheld Echocardiography in Clinical Management

HHE assisted with the initial evaluation of LV function, bioprosthetic aortic valve and function, presence of calcific mixed mitral valve disease, and dilated right ventricle with pressure overload.

Final Diagnosis

The diagnosis was severe bioprosthetic aortic valve stenosis from structural valve degeneration (SVD) with severe calcific mitral valve stenosis and pulmonary hypertension.

Teaching Point

- There has been an increased use of aortic bioprosthesis compared with mechanical prosthesis. The 2017 focused update of the American College of Cardiology (ACC)/American Heart Association (AHA) guidelines, suggests that it is reasonable (class IIa) to implant bioprostheses in patients >70 years old.

- The goal at the time of valve implant in the aortic position is for the valve to outlive the patient; however, biological valves are prone to structural valve deterioration (SVD) over time.[1]
- There is no consensus on the definition of SVD. The 2016 European Association of Cardiovascular Imaging guidelines[2] suggest defining SVD as: (1) an increase in mean gradient ≥10 mm Hg (possible SVD) or ≥20 mm Hg (significant SVD) during follow up, with a concomitant decrease in effective orifice area (EOA) and abnormal valve leaflet morphology and mobility; and/or (2) new onset or worsening of prosthetic regurgitation.
- The Valve Academic Research Consortium-2 recommendations[3] suggest consideration of valve dysfunction at follow up if there is an increase in the mean gradient >10 mm Hg, a decrease in the EOA of >0.3 to 0.4 cm^2, or a reduction in the dimensionless velocity index of >0.1 to 0.13 from the echocardiography performed within 30 days after transcatheter aortic valve replacement (TAVR).
- Morphologic changes of leaflet thickening, calcification, flail, pannus and/or reduced or increased mobility from avulsion compared with the baseline echocardiography performed at 1 to 3 months after the procedure suggest SVD.
- Causes of SVD manifests as calcification and leaflet degradation leading to valve stenosis or leaflet tear with ensuing valve regurgitation. Bovine pericardial valves have a greater propensity to develop stenosis, whereas porcine valves have a tendency to develop leaflet tear with regurgitation.
- Valve degeneration appears more rapidly on the left-sided cardiac valves than on the low-pressure right-sided cardiac valves and in the mitral valve more rapidly than in the aortic position. In older adults the longevity of bioprosthetic valves in the aortic position is between 10 to 20 years; and in the mitral position, 8 to 15 years. Younger age and increased BMI are associated with a more rapid SVD.
- The treatment for SVD has conventionally been surgical valve replacement; however, because of age and comorbidities in this cohort, redo surgery is associated with increased morbidity and mortality. Valve-in-valve replacement by TAVR has become a feasible option in such patients.

References

1. Rodriguez-Gabella T, Voisine P, Puri R, Pibarot P, Rodés-Cabau J. Aortic bioprosthetic valve durability: incidence, mechanisms, predictors, and management of surgical and transcatheter valve degeneration. *J Am Coll Cardiol.* 2017;70(8):1013–1028.
2. Lancellotti P, Pibarot P, Chambers J, et al. Recommendations for the imaging assessment of prosthetic heart valves: a report from the European Association of Cardiovascular Imaging endorsed by the Chinese Society of Echocardiography, the Interamerican Society of Echocardiography and the Brazilian Department of Cardiovascular Imaging. *Eur Heart J Cardiovasc Imaging.* 2016;17:589–590.
3. Kappetein AP, Head SJ, Généreux P, et al. Updated standardized endpoint definitions for transcatheter aortic valve implantation: The Valve Academic Research Consortium-2 consensus document. *J Am Coll Cardiol.* 2012;60:1438–1454.

Case 2—A 65-Year-Old Man With Dyspnea Status Post TAVR and TMVR

History

Cardiology was consulted by the ICU team for worsening dyspnea on exertion and pedal edema of recent onset in a 65-year-old man with a history of severe aortic stenosis and mitral regurgitation (MR), who had undergone TAVR with a 29-mm Sapien valve (Edwards Lifesciences, Irvine, California) a year ago and percutaneous mitral valve repair (TMVR) with two mitral clips (MC) for a flail A2 scallop of anterior mitral leaflet 6 months before presentation.

Past Medical History

The patient has had two previous failed renal transplants and is currently on dialysis three times per week. He also had hypertension, atrial fibrillation, recurrent deep venous thrombosis, chronic pulmonary emboli maintained on chronic anticoagulation, a chronic inferior vena cava filter, squamous cell carcinoma at the site of AV fistula status post resection, and colostomy secondary to colectomy for diverticulitis.

Physical Examination

A pulmonary artery catheter was in place with a pulmonary artery pressure of 64/30 mm Hg. There was a 2/6 apical holosystolic murmur and a 2/6 ejection systolic murmur at the right second intercostal space.

Laboratory Values

N-terminal proB-type natriuretic peptide (NT-proBNP) was 52,000 pg/mL (normal 89 pg/mL)

Electrocardiography

ECG showed atrial fibrillation with controlled ventricular response (Fig. 11.9).

Chest Radiography

CXR showed two mitral clips, a Sapien valve bioprosthesis cardiomegaly and pulmonary artery catheter (Fig. 11.10).

Transesophageal Echocardiography Review

TEE performed during the previous mitral clip implant was reviewed. It showed a double mitral inflow on either side of the two central mitral clips at the end of the procedure. Mitral regurgitation (MR) severity decreased from severe to mild, with an eccentric jet anterolateral to the clips and an effective orifice area (EOA) of 0.11 cm² and regurgitant volume of 16 mL consistent with mild MR. Mean mitral valve gradient after mitral clip implant was 5 mm Hg at a heart rate of 85 bpm.

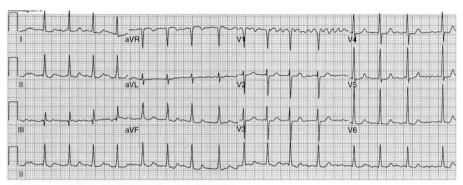

Fig. 11.9   ECG showing atrial fibrillation with controlled ventricular response and non specific ST changes.

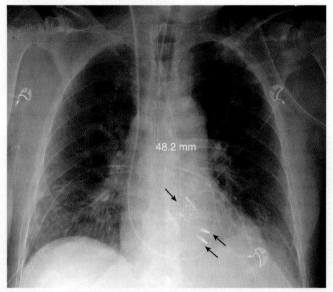

Fig. 11.10   Portable CXR showing mild cardiomegaly, mild pulmonary edema, Sapien transcatheter aortic valve (red arrow) and two mitral clips (black arrows) in place and pulmonary arterial catheter.

Handheld Echocardiography

HHE was done at the bedside during initial consultation and showed normal left ventricular size and systolic function, a 29-mm Sapien valve in the appropriate location and at an appropriate height, and mitral clips in place with mild-to-moderate enlargement of the right ventricular outflow tract (Fig. 11.11, Video 11.4). There was mild-to-moderate anterior aortic paravalvular leak (PVL) in the parasternal long-axis (Fig. 11.12A) and short-axis (Fig. 11.12B) views. A mild posterior PVL was also seen. There were two central mitral clips with double orifice mitral valve (Figs. 11.13 and 11.14A, Video 11.5) and residual prolapse lateral to the clip with a significant MR jet originating at the site of the residual leaflet prolapse lateral to the clips (Fig. 11.14B, Video 11.6).

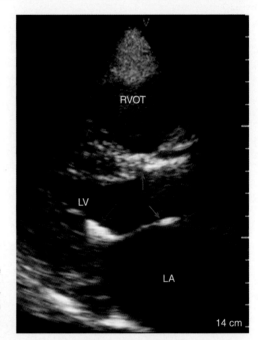

Fig. 11.11 HHE PLAX view showing mitral valve clips in proper position (red arrow) and appropriately positioned Sapien aortic valve stent (yellow arrows). There is enlargement of the left atrium (LA) and right ventricular outflow tract (RVOT). *LV,* Left ventricle.

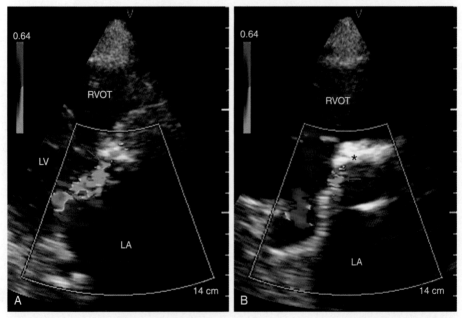

Fig. 11.12 (A) HHE PLAX view with color Doppler showing mild-to-moderate anterior paravalvular leak (yellow arrow). Both the left atrium (LA) and right ventricular outflow tract are dilated. (B) HHE SAX view with color Doppler of the Sapien aortic valve showing paravalvular leak originating at 9 to 11 o'clock position (yellow arrow) (assuming aortic stent [black asterisk] as a clock with 12 o'clock at the top of the stent). Both the LA and right ventricular outflow tract (RVOT) are dilated. *LV,* Left ventricle; *RV,* right ventricle.

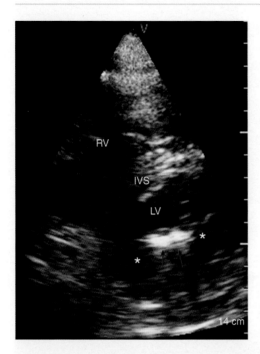

Fig. 11.13 HHE SAX view at the mitral valve level showing two mitral clips in the center (red arrows) and a double-orifice mitral valve (white asterisks). Mild flattening of the interventricular septum is present because of pulmonary hypertension. *IVS,* Interventricular septum; *LV,* left ventricle; *RV,* right ventricle.

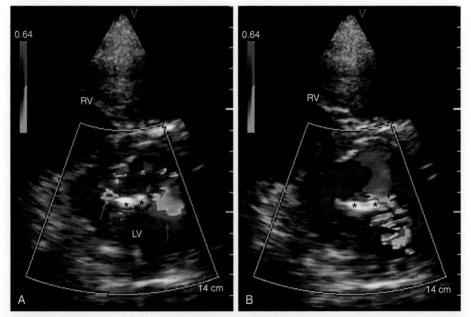

Fig. 11.14 (A) HHE SAX view with color Doppler in diastole showing flow across the double-orifice mitral valve (yellow arrows) with clips in the center (black asterisks). (B) HHE SAX view with color Doppler in systole showing moderate-appearing residual MR (red arrows) lateral to the clips (black asterisks). *LV,* Left ventricle; *RV,* right ventricle.

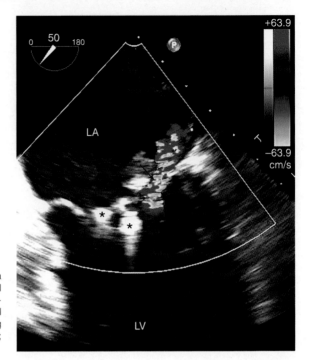

Fig. 11.15 TEE bicommissural view at a 50-degree angle showing two central mitral clips (black asterisks) with residual moderate-to-severe eccentric mitral regurgitation jet (red arrow) originating lateral to the lateral clip. *LA,* Left atrium; *LV,* left ventricle.

Subsequent Hospital Course

A TEE was subsequently performed and confirmed a moderate-to-severe MR jet anterolateral to the lateral clip on color Doppler (Fig. 11.15) and moderate-appearing aortic PVL (Fig. 11.16). A diagnosis of moderate-to-severe hemodynamically significant recurrent MR lateral to the lateral clip was made. The patient underwent a third clip deployment successfully. Postoperatively he required aggressive dialysis; and after a prolonged hospital stay, he was discharged home.

Utility of HHE in Clinical Management

HHE demonstrated both the residual MR location and severity and the etiology of regurgitation caused by residual or new MV prolapse. HHE also showed severity and location of aortic paravalvular regurgitation, thereby expediting diagnostic workup.

Final Diagnosis

Recurrent MR secondary to residual mitral valve prolapse and mild to moderate PVL after TAVR and TMVR with mitral clips in a 65-year-old man with multiple comorbidities.

Teaching Point

TRANSCATHETER AORTIC VALVE REPLACEMENT (TAVR) AND PERCUTANEOUS MITRAL VALVE REPAIR USING MITRAL CLIP

- Aortic valve stenosis (AS) mainly affects elderly patients and has a poor prognosis after symptoms of dyspnea, angina, or syncope occur. Surgical aortic valve replacement (sAVR)

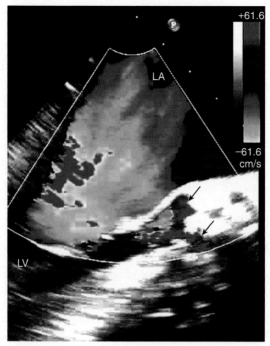

Fig. 11.16 TEE color Doppler long-axis view in diastole showing moderate anterior and posterior aortic paravalvular regurgitation (black arrow). *LA,* Left atrium; *LV,* left ventricle.

has been the gold-standard treatment; but, with an ageing and an increasingly comorbid population, the need for less invasive therapies was identified because many such patients do not get referred for sAVR.

- TAVR was first performed in 2002 in a human patient.
- TAVR is a safe and effective treatment for patients with symptomatic severe aortic stenosis at intermediate, high, and prohibitive surgical risk. With the expansion of TAVR and eligibility of lower-risk patients, management of procedure-related complications is increasingly important, along with a focus on longer-term outcomes. Common complications of TAVR include vascular complications, bleeding, residual PVL, and new-onset conduction disturbances. Recent changes to the valve design limit the depth of the valve frame in left ventricular outflow tract (LVOT) during deployment, reducing the interaction of the valve with the LVOT and conduction system. The new design also includes a skirt at the bottom of the valve frame, which has reduced the incidence of PVL to <2%. The incidence of conduction abnormalities is higher with the self-expanding valve that the balloon-expandable valve.
- Greater-than-mild PVL is associated with an adverse outcome. PVL quantitation is semi-quantitative. PVL is graded based on the number and size of regurgitant jets, vena contracta width of the jets, and circumferential extent of the jets around the valve frame. Color Doppler regurgitation assessment of PVL in a patient after TAVR requires multiple parasternal and apical views and off-angle views to characterize origin and severity of PVL.
- Doppler evaluation includes diastolic flow reversal in the descending aorta by color Doppler and PW Doppler, aortic insufficiency (AI) jet density on CW Doppler, and pressure half time of the AI jet. A comprehensive standard echocardiography is used to quantify valve regurgitation severity.[1]

- Randomized trial data on the benefit of TMVR with mitral clips in patients after TAVR is lacking, and the treatment approach is individualized. Postprocedure ≥2+ MR, and not preprocedure MR severity, was associated with increased cardiovascular morbidity and mortality and adverse LV and RV remodeling.[2]
- TMVR is a novel alternative treatment option for patients with severe MR who are at high risk for conventional mitral valve surgery or are inoperable. Currently TMVR with mitral clips (Abbott Laboratories, USA) is the only clinically approved procedure in the United States.
- Compared with surgical mitral valve repair, TMVR is less effective at reducing MR, and residual MR is commonly observed after TMVR.[3]
- In the EVEREST trial in which patients with significant MR were randomized to surgical repair or TMVR with mitral clip procedure, the mitral valve repair procedural failure was defined as unsuccessful mitral clip implantation or residual MR of 3+/4+. This was observed in approximately 10% of patients who underwent TMVR and was associated with adverse clinical outcomes.[3]
- Residual MR 2+ after TMVR might be associated with poor prognosis in high-risk patients such as those with LVEF ≤40%, chronic renal insufficiency, and NYHA-class IV heart failure.
- Presence of mitral clip and reduction in mitral valve area after clip deployment makes residual MR quantitation more challenging than in a native valve. Residual MR jet area relative to left atrial area (for central jets), number of residual MR jets, measurable vena contracta width of MR jet/s, 3D vena contracta area (central and eccentric jets), and pulmonary vein Doppler pattern are used to assess residual MR severity.

References

1. Pibarot P, Hahn RT, Weissman NJ, Monaghan MJ. Assessment of paravalvular regurgitation following TAVR: a proposal of unifying grading scheme. *JACC Cardiovasc Imaging*. 2015;8(3):340–360.
2. Ben-Assa E, Biner S, Banai S, et al. Clinical impact of post procedural mitral regurgitation after transcatheter aortic valve replacement. *Int J Cardiol*. 2020;299:215–221. Available at: https://doi.org/10.1016/j.ijcard.2019.07.092.
3. Feldman T., Foster E., Glower D., et al. Percutaneous repair or surgery for mitral regurgitation. *N Engl J Med*. 2011;364:1395–1406.

Case 3—An 86-Year-Old Man Post TAVR Presents With Dyspnea

History

An 86-year-old man status post TAVR at an outside facility 3 months ago, presented with dyspnea on exertion and, more recently, at rest and increasing bilateral ankle swelling.

Physical Examination

There was a visible "CV" wave in the internal jugular vein. There was 4/6 holosystolic apical and left lower para-sternal murmur and a 1/6 ejection systolic murmur at the right second intercostal space.

Laboratory Values

N-terminal proB-type natriuretic peptide (NT-proBNP) was 6058 pg/mL (<450 pg/mL)

Electrocardiography

ECG showed atrial fibrillation with controlled ventricular response.

Chest Radiography

CXR showed cardiomegaly with bilateral pulmonary venous congestion.

Handheld Echocardiography

A Sapien valve with the stent edges in the LV outflow tract at appropriate depth was seen in the aortic position (Fig. 11.17). There was severe left atrial enlargement and marked enlargement of the right ventricular outflow tract (RVOT) with moderate-to-severely reduced function (Figs. 11.17-11.19, Video 11.7). Color Doppler interrogation revealed nonturbulent flow into the aortic valve with trivial anterior paravalvular leak, calcification of the anterior mitral leaflet, and moderate posteriorly directed mitral regurgitation jet. Short-axis view at the aortic valve level showed severe biatrial enlargement, dilated and hypokinetic RVOT, and normal-appearing AV stent and AV leaflet motion to the extent visualized (Fig. 11.18). Color Doppler showed trivial paravalvular leak visible in the short-axis view (Fig. 11.19, Video 11.7). RV inflow view showed severe RV and RA enlargement and color Doppler showed severe tricuspid regurgitation (Fig. 11.20, Video 11.8). Apical four-chamber view showed four-chamber enlargement with marked biatrial enlargement. The right ventricle was moderately dilated. There was moderately reduced left ventricular systolic function and mild mitral annular calcification (Fig. 11.21, Video 11.9). Color Doppler in the apical four-chamber view showed moderate central mitral regurgitation and severe tricuspid regurgitation (TR) (Fig. 11.22). Diffuse left ventricular hypo-kinesis without regional wall motion abnormalities were seen in the four-chamber (Fig. 11.21, Video 11.9) and two-chamber views. Subcostal view demonstrated markedly dilated inferior vena cava (IVC) with severely blunted inspiratory collapse and dilated hepatic vein (Fig. 11.23).

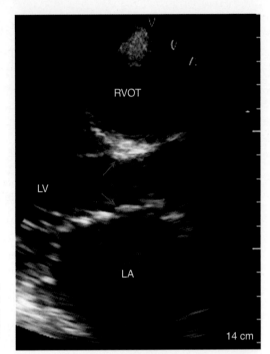

Fig. 11.17 HHE PLAX view showing the Sapien valve stent edges in the left ventricle (LV) outflow tract (yellow arrow). Also shown are severe left atrial enlargement and marked enlargement of right ventricular outflow tract (RVOT). *LA*, Left atrium.

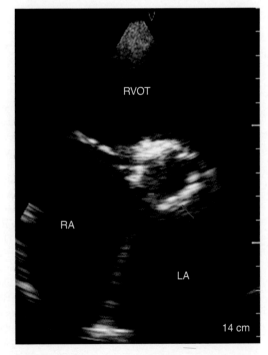

Fig. 11.18 HHE parasternal short-axis view at the base showing Sapien valve circular stent (yellow arrow). Also shown are severe biatrial enlargement and dilated RVOT. *LA*, Left atrium; *RA*, right atrium; *RVOT*, right ventricular outflow tract.

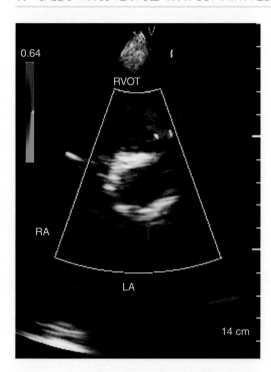

Fig. 11.19 HHE color Doppler parasternal short-axis view at the base in diastole showing a Sapien aortic valve stent in the center (yellow arrow). There is mild pulmonic valve insufficiency (red arrow). Also shown are severe bi-atrial enlargement and dilated RVOT. *LA,* Left atrium; *RA,* right atrium; *RVOT,* right ventricular outflow tract.

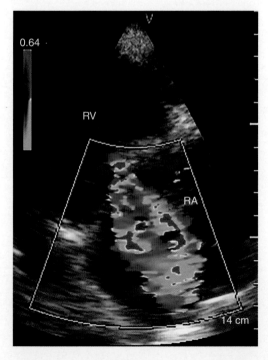

Fig. 11.20 HHE color Doppler right ventricle (RV) inflow view showing markedly dilated right atrium (RA) and RV and blue mosaic jet of severe tricuspid regurgitation at a normal aliasing velocity of 0.64 m/s.

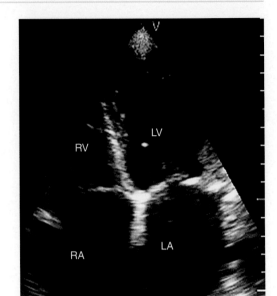

Fig. 11.21 HHE apical 4-chamber view showing marked biatrial enlargement, moderate right ventricular and mild left ventricular enlargement. *LA,* Left atrium; *LV,* left ventricle; *RA,* right atrium; *RV,* right ventricle.

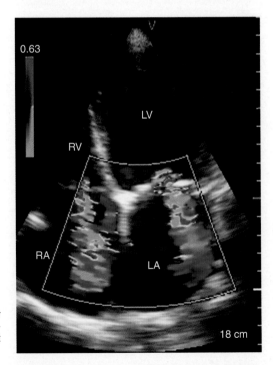

Fig. 11.22 HHE color Doppler apical 4-chamber showing significant mitral and tricuspid regurgitation. *LA,* Left atrium; *LV,* left ventricle; *RA,* right atrium; *RV,* right ventricle.

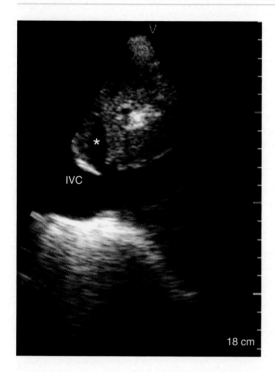

Fig. 11.23 HHE subcostal view showing a markedly dilated inferior vena cava (IVC) and dilated hepatic vein (white asterisk). There was minimal respiratory collapse of the IVC indicating right atrial pressure of 15 mm Hg.

Hospital Course

A diagnosis of congestive heart failure with biventricular dysfunction, volume overload and significant MR and TR was made. Jugular venous distention and pedal edema were secondary to severe RV dysfunction and CV neck vein wave from severe TR and severely elevated right atrial pressure. Patient was given intravenous diuretics followed by oral diuresis and discharged home on continued diuretics.

Utility of HHE in Clinical Management

HHE demonstrated a normally functioning Sapien valve in the aortic position. It also demonstrated severe RV and RA enlargement, severe tricuspid regurgitation, and moderate mitral regurgitation with severe biatrial enlargement and increased RA pressure. It also confirmed the etiology of the patient's dyspnea being related to elevated filling pressures and mitral and tricuspid regurgitation.

Final Diagnosis

The diagnosis was heart failure exacerbation caused by RV dysfunction, severe TR, and significant MR in an 86-year-old man after TAVR.

Teaching Point

Significant TR is a common finding in TAVR candidates, and TR frequently improves after TAVR. However, the presence of atrial fibrillation in the presence of significant TR usually indicates a lack of significant improvement of TR after TAVR. RV size and function are more important predictors of outcome after TAVR than TR severity before TAVR.[1] Patients with significant residual MR or

TR post TAVR demonstrate a strong trend toward higher mortality after TAVR. Therefore a thorough evaluation of the mechanisms underlying concomitant mitral and tricuspid valve regurgitation should be performed to determine the aortic valve implantation (TAVI)-related futility.[2]

In a meta-analysis of nine studies among 27,614 patients who underwent TAVR between 2011 and 2018, mortality was twice as high at short-term, mid-term, and long-term follow-up among 6255 patients with significant tricuspid regurgitation in the group.[1]

In one study, among the 1110 patients undergoing TAVR, 177 had significant MR. These patients had a 3-fold higher all-cause mortality at 6 months (35% vs 10.2%), as well as cardiac mortality (20.9% vs 6%) compared with patients without significant MR. MR severity improved in 60% of patients after TAVR. A mitral annular diameter of more than 35.5 mm and calcification severity by multidetector computed tomography were independent predictors of persistent MR after TAVR.[3] The presence of significant MR and TR should be included in the evaluation and decision-making process among patients who are TAVR candidates.

References

1. Narut P, Veraprapas K, Nithi T, et al. Baseline significant tricuspid regurgitation is associated with higher mortality in transcatheter aortic valve replacement. systemic review and meta-analysis. *J Cardiovasc Med.* 2019;20(7):4786.
2. Schwartz LA, Rozenbaum Z, Ghantous E, et al. Impact of right ventricular dysfunction and tricuspid regurgitation on outcomes in patients undergoing transcatheter aortic valve replacement. *J Am Soc Echocardiogr.* 2017;30(1):36–46.
3. Cortés C, Amat-Santos IJ, Nombela-Franco L, et al. Mitral regurgitation after transcatheter aortic valve replacement. *JACC Cardiovasc Interv.* 2016;9(15):1603–1614.

CHAPTER 12

Case 1—A 72-Year-Old Man With Fatigue After Mitral Valve Replacement

History

A 72-year-old man status post pericardial mitral valve (MV) replacement for a flail mitral valve and severe mitral regurgitation, Cox maze procedure for paroxysmal atrial fibrillation, and left atrial appendage ligation 10 days ago, presented with symptoms of fatigue, pleuritic precordial chest pain, intermittent blurred vision, and possible facial droop.

A brain MRI showed small new subacute cerebral infarcts, which appeared to have occurred perioperatively for MV replacement with no acute ischemic changes, and the patient was admitted under neurology service.

Cardiology was consulted for atrial fibrillation after admission and for anticoagulation guidance.

Pre-MV replacement surgery coronary angiogram had shown minimal nonobstructive coronary artery disease with 10% to 20% stenosis.

Physical Examination

Blood pressure was 100/60 mm Hg. There was no focal neurologic sign. Heart sounds were muffled. There was no pericardial rub or new murmur.

Laboratory Values

Hemoglobin was 10.3 g/dL, creatinine was 0.85 mg/dL.

Electrocardiography

ECG showed atrial fibrillation with controlled ventricular response and low voltage (Fig. 12.1). International normalized ratio (INR) was 2.1 and 2.3 over the last 24 hours.

Chest Radiography

CXR (Fig. 12.2) showed significant cardiomegaly and bilateral pulmonary venous congestion compared with predischarge CXR.

Handheld Echocardiography

A bedside HHE showed a new moderate pericardial effusion posterolateral to LV and small effusion anterior to RV in the parasternal long-axis view (Fig. 12.3). Effusion was moderate-to-large posterolateral to the LV in the apical three-chamber view and showed a few pericardial strands (Fig. 12.4, Video 12.1). The effusion was new compared with the predischarge echocardiogram

137

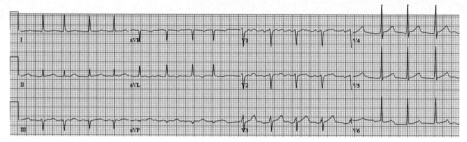

Fig. 12.1   One-lead ECG showing atrial fibrillation with heart rate of 100 bpm and slightly reduced voltage.

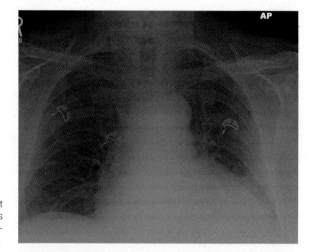

Fig. 12.2 CXR showing significant cardiomegaly and pulmonary venous congestion. Cardiac silhouette had increased since last predischarge CXR.

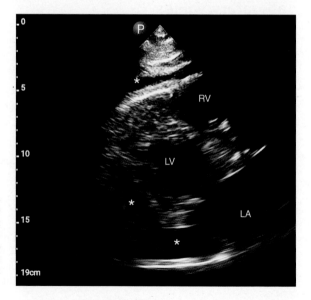

Fig. 12.3 HHE parasternal long-axis view showing moderate pericardial effusion posterolateral to the left ventricle (white asterisks) and small effusion anterior to the right ventricle (small white asterisk). *LA*, Left atrium; *LV*, left ventricle; *RV*, right ventricle.

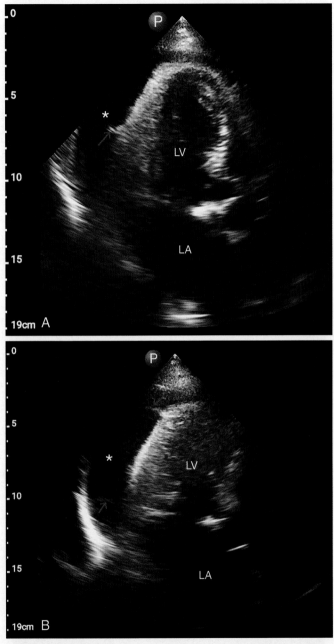

Fig. 12.4   (A) HHE apical 3-chamber end-systolic view showing normal left ventricle (LV) size and function with normal endocardial thickening, a dilated left atrium (LA), and a moderate-to-large pericardial effusion predominantly posterolateral to the left ventricle (white asterisk). (B) HHE off-axis apical 3-chamber view to show the pericardial effusion, which appears slightly larger in this view. Pericardial strands (yellow arrows) are shown.

done 1 week ago. LV and RV function (Video 12.1) and bioprosthetic MV function were normal with no central or perivalvular regurgitation. The inferior vena cava (IVC) was not dilated and showed normal inspiratory collapse.

Standard Echocardiography

A subsequent standard echocardiogram confirmed a moderate-to-large pericardial effusion, with the largest fluid collection posterolateral to the LV and a small anterior effusion (Fig. 12.5, Video 12.2). LV and RV function and bioprosthetic valve function were normal (Fig. 12.6, Video 12.2). Mean MV gradient was 5 mm Hg. There was no diastolic RV or RA chamber collapse or significant mitral or tricuspid respiratory variation; however, atrial fibrillation with a HR of 100 to 120 bpm made evaluation of tamponade physiology difficult. Peak pulmonary artery pressure was 30 mm Hg.

Clinical Course

As a result of the need for continued anticoagulation and the risk for an increase in size of the pericardial effusion, new-onset atrial fibrillation likely caused by pericardial inflammation, and borderline low blood pressures, a decision was made to perform pericardiocentesis after holding one dose of coumadin.

440 cc of bloody fluid was removed after which the pigtail catheter was placed and removed 48 hours later.

CXR after pericardiocentesis showed a reduction in cardiac silhouette and an improvement in pulmonary venous congestion.

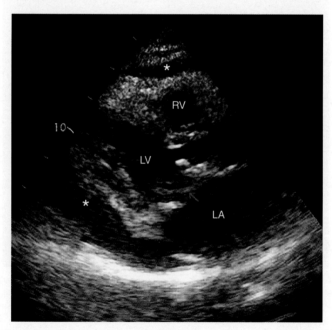

Fig. 12.5 Standard echocardiogram parasternal long-axis view showing moderate pericardial effusion posterolateral to the left ventricle (LV) (white asterisk) and small effusion anterior to the right ventricle (RV) (white asterisk). A bioprosthetic mitral valve is seen (yellow arrow). *LA,* Left atrium.

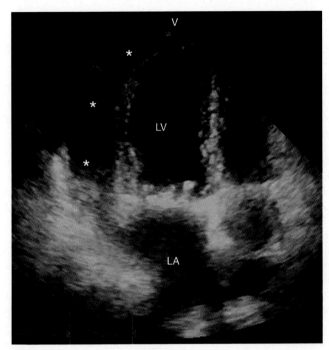

Fig. 12.6   Standard echocardiogram apical 4-chamber view showing a moderate-to-large pericardial effusion (white asterisks) lateral to the left ventricle. *LA*, Left atrium; *LV*, left ventricle.

The patient was started on oral amiodarone and low-dose metoprolol. He had an uneventful course and was discharged after attaining therapeutic INR subsequent to removal of pericardial catheter.

The patient was doing well at the 2-week follow up. Hemoglobin was 12.3, and CXR was unremarkable.

Utility of Handheld Echocardiography in Patient Management

HHE allowed for a rapid assessment for the etiology of fatigue and new atrial fibrillation caused by pericardial effusion. It showed normal LV function during atrial fibrillation and normal bioprosthetic mitral valve function.

Final Diagnosis

Inflammatory pericardial effusion after mitral valve replacement precipitating atrial fibrillation and fatigue was the diagnosis. Neurologic symptoms were likely secondary to cerebral hypoperfusion.

Teaching Point

The normal pericardium is a fibroserous sac comprising of an outer, thicker, fibrous layer (the parietal pericardium) and a thin, inner, serous layer (the visceral pericardium). The pericardial sac contains approximately 25 mL of fluid and is ≤2 mm thick.[1]

Transthoracic echocardiogram (TTE) is the first-line imaging modality to evaluate patients with potential cardiovascular symptomatology after cardiac surgery.

Pericardial effusion is common after cardiac surgery because of postoperative pericarditis and may increase in size and lead to cardiac tamponade in some patients if untreated. Pericardial inflammation may trigger atrial fibrillation.

Pericardial effusion can be trivial-to-large and localized, loculated, or circumferential. As a general guide it can be graded as trivial when pericardial fluid is present only in systole; small, <1 cm (50–100 mL); moderate, 1 to 2 cm (100–500 mL); large, >2 cm (>500 mL); very large, >2.5 cm (Fig. 12.7).

Intrapericardial fibrinous strands suggest either an inflammatory etiology or clotted blood. Two-dimensional (2D) echocardiogram helps diagnose the presence and amount of pericardial effusion, focal vs generalized effusion, and if there are features of cardiac tamponade. These include right atrial and right ventricular diastolic collapse, elevated right atrial pressure assessed by evaluating the IVC, and hepatic vein size by 2D echocardiogram. The M-mode feature also available in some HHE systems allow M-mode assessment of interventricular dependence.

Other Doppler features of tamponade such as changes in mitral and tricuspid inflow velocities by PW Doppler require a standard echocardiogram at present, because spectral Doppler features are not available in most HHE systems. With tamponade there is an exaggerated decrease in LV cavity size and in mitral inflow velocities during the inspiratory phase of the respiratory cycle; whereas with expiration there is an increase in LV cavity size, as well as mitral inflow velocities. The opposite changes occur on RV and tricuspid inflow. Expiratory hepatic vein diastolic Doppler

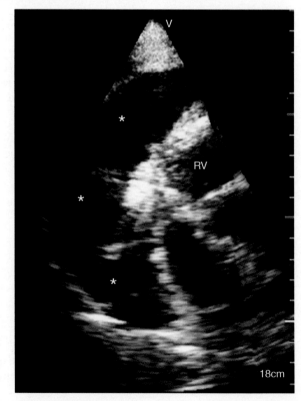

Fig. 12.7 HHE nonstandard view performed immediately before pericardiocentesis to show the largest size of the pericardial effusion in another patient with cardiac tamponade from a large pericardial effusion (white asterisks). *RV,* Right ventricle.

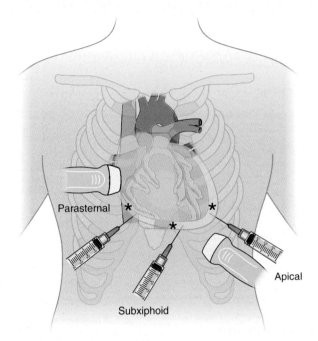

Fig. 12.8 Diagram showing transducer and needle positioning for pericardiocentesis in the subxiphoid, apical, and parasternal windows. The needle positioning and direction is determined by the position and angulation of the ultrasound transducer showing the largest pericardial effusion. Ultrasound imaging during pericardiocentesis is also used to confirm placement of the needle in the pericardial space by injection of and subsequent visualization of saline contrast bubbles in the pericardial space.

velocity reversal is a specific sign of pericardial tamponade. The essential physiology behind interventricular dependence is the inability of the LV free wall to expand during diastole and dissociation between intrathoracic and cardiac pressure. An inspiratory decrease in intrathoracic pressure pulls blood into the vena cava, and an expiratory increase in intrathoracic pressure increases pulmonary venous return to the left atrium. An inspiratory increase in RV inflow pushes the septum toward the LV, and an expiratory increase in LV inflow pushes the IVS toward the RV. Because RV end-diastolic pressure increases markedly during end expiration, the TV gets closed and right atrial contraction in late diastole results in expiratory late-diastolic hepatic vein flow reversal.

Echocardiography helps determine the best site for pericardiocentesis by identifying the site of the largest pericardial fluid collection (Fig. 12.7), helps confirm entry into the pericardial space by visualization of the needle, and helps further confirmation by injection of saline contrast bubbles after aspiration of an equivalent amount of fluid. Parasternal, apical, and subxiphoid approaches are used for pericardiocentesis (Fig. 12.8). Bedside HHE in particular is readily available, portable and bedside, safe, and can be performed in urgent situations.

References

1. Klein AL, Abbara S, Agler DA, et al. American Society of Echocardiography clinical recommendations for multimodality cardiovascular imaging of patients with pericardial disease: Endorsed by the Society for Cardiovascular Magnetic Resonance and society of cardiovascular computed tomography. *J Am Soc Echocardiogr.* 2013;26:965–1012.e15.

CHAPTER 13

Case 1—Cardiology Consult Before Noncardiac Surgery for Brain Tumor

History

A 72-year-old Caucasian woman presented with a recent onset of headaches and visual changes and was found to have two cerebral tumors with surrounding edema in the right parietal and occipital lobes on brain MRI.

There was a history of colon adenocarcinoma surgery 4 years ago.

Cardiology was consulted by neurosurgery for cardiac clearance for brain surgery due to two consecutive troponin levels of 37 and 47 over a 24-hour period (n ≤ 10 ng/L) and a cardiac murmur. There was no prior cardiac history and no history of chest pain during current admission.

Physical Examination

Patient's functional capacity was >4 metabolic equivalents (METS). There was a 2/6 ejection systolic murmur over the right second intercostal space.

Laboratory Values

Serum creatinine was 1.9 mg/dL (normal <1.04) and had been increasing over the last 2 days.

Brain MRI

Brain MRI showed a large right parietal lobe mass (Fig. 13.1).

Electrocardiography

ECG (Fig. 13.2) showed the voltage criteria for left ventricular hypertrophy, and nonspecific ST changes were likely related to repolarization abnormality.

Handheld Echocardiography

Bedside HHE during cardiac consultation showed hyperkinetic left ventricular wall motion and systolic function without regional wall motion abnormality shown in the 4-chamber (Figs. 13.3 and 13.4, Videos 13.1 and 13.2) and 3-chamber (Figs. 13.5A-B and 13.6) views. It also showed mild increases in intraventricular flow velocities as evident by turbulent blood flow in the left ventricular outflow tract (Figs. 13.4 and 13.6, Video 13.2). Valve function was normal on two-dimensional (2D) and color Doppler. Subcostal views showed normal trileaflet aortic, tricuspid, and pulmonic valves (Fig. 13.7) and a normal inferior vena cava (IVC).

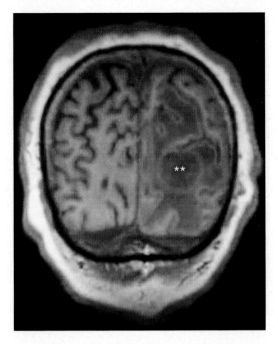

Fig. 13.1 Brain MRI showing a large parietal lobe mass (double white asterisks).

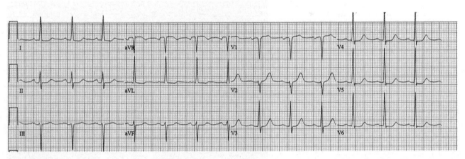

Fig. 13.2 12 lead EG showing voltage criteria for left ventricular hypertrophy and nonspecific ST changes in lateral leads likely related to repolarization abnormality.

Hospital Course

Troponin leak was thought to be secondary to renal insufficiency causing reduced renal clearance and contribution from left ventricular hypertrophy with a relative increase in heart rate and left ventricular (LV) hyperkinesis leading to a myocardial supply-demand mismatch. Subarachnoid hemorrhage can cause troponin elevation with reversible wall motion abnormalities.

Based on HHE findings and low clinical risk score, the patient was cleared for surgery after starting beta-blocker to aim for a heart rate of 60 to 70 bpm and reduce LV hyperkinesis and IV fluids to reduce intraventricular gradient and for pre-renal azotemia. Patient underwent surgery without complications, and biopsy confirmed metastatic colon adenocarcinoma. Postoperative course was uneventful and she received outpatient radiation therapy for brain tumor metastasis.

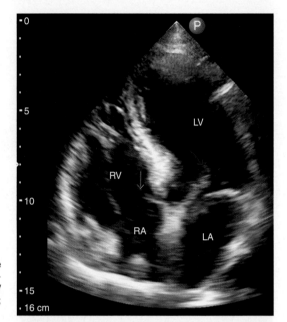

Fig. 13.3   HHE apical 4-chamber diastole view with open mitral (red arrow) and tricuspid (yellow arrow) valves and normal LV shape. *LA*, Left atrium; *LV*, left ventricle; *RA*, right atrium; *RV*, right ventricle.

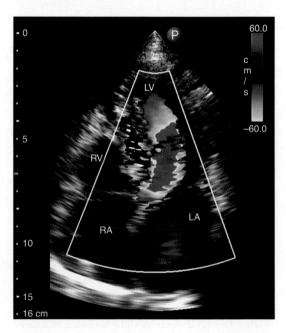

Fig. 13.4   HHE apical 4-chamber color Doppler view showing turbulent flow in the mid left ventricle (LV) cavity as the etiology of systolic murmur from a hyperkinetic LV with increased intraventricular flow velocities. There is no tricuspid or mitral regurgitation. *LA*, Left atrium; *RA*, right atrium; *RV*, right ventricle.

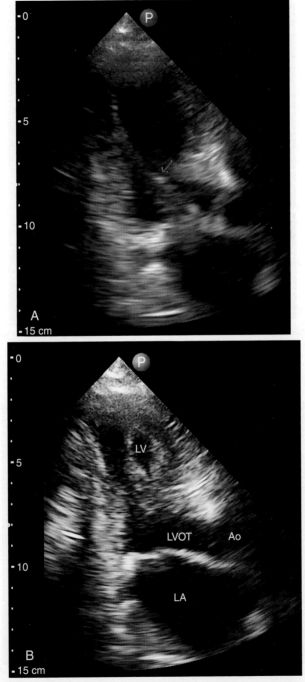

Fig. 13.5 (A) HHE apical 3-chamber end-diastole view showing prominent left ventricle (LV) chord in close proximity to a sigmoid interventricular septum (yellow arrow). (B) HHE apical 3-chamber end-systolic view showing LV cavity obliteration and chordal septal contact. There is left atrial enlargement. *Ao,* Aortic root; *LA,* left atrium; *LVOT,* left ventricular outflow tract.

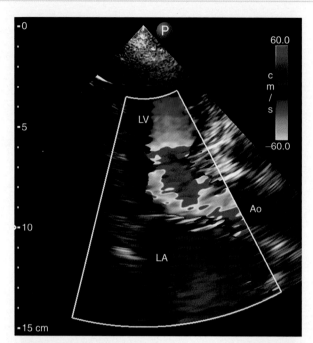

Fig. 13.6   HHE apical 3-chamber color Doppler view in systole showing turbulent flow in the mid left ventricle (LV) from a hyperkinetic LV as the etiology of systolic murmur. *Ao*, Aortic root; *LA*, left atrium.

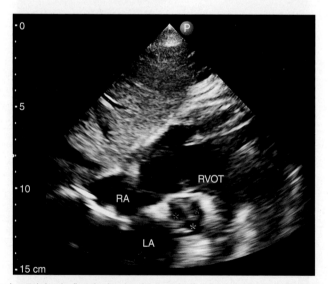

Fig. 13.7   HHE subcostal view in diastole showing right ventricular inflow with the open tricuspid valve leaflets and outflow. A normal trileaflet aortic valve in the closed position noncoronary (red asterisk), left coronary (yellow asterisk), and right coronary cusps (blue asterisk) is shown. Both atria are shown with the interatrial septum between them and with left atrial enlargement. HHE technology is able to provide assessment of cardiac structures including valves. *LA*, Left atrium; *RA*, right atrium; *RVOT*, right ventricular outflow tract.

Teaching Point

PERIOPERATIVE CARDIAC RISK ASSESSMENT

- The purpose of cardiovascular perioperative cardiac risk assessment is to evaluate the benefits and risks of the surgery and optimize the timing of the surgery.
- Information obtained from the history, physical examination, ECG, and type of surgery is obtained to develop an initial estimate of perioperative cardiac risk.

RISK MODELS

- Revised cardiac risk index (RCRI). This score uses six risk factors: high-risk surgery (e.g., vascular surgery), history of ischemic heart disease, heart failure, cerebrovascular disease, diabetes mellitus, and serum creatinine >2 mg/dL. It is used to predict the risk of cardiac death, nonfatal myocardial infarction, and nonfatal cardiac arrest based on the number of patient has. No risk factors, 0.4%; one risk factor, 1%; two risk factors, 2.4%; and three or more risk factors, 5.4%.
- The American College of Surgeons National Surgical Quality Improvement Program (NSQIP) risk calculator, http://riskcalculator.facs.org/RiskCalculator/.

Role of HHE in Care Delivery

Allowed assessment of etiology of systolic murmur and confirmed no significant myocardial or valvular heart disease prior to brain surgery.

INDEX

Page numbers followed by *f* indicates figures and *t* indicates tables.